Side-Swiped

My Journey with Peritoneal Cancer;

When The Unexpected Happens

by

Nora Kirlew Hampden

Dedicated to:

The memory of my mother, Sarah A. Kirlew, who raised me to love and trust the Lord.

My sons, Winston and Jason for their love and belief in me despite the odds.

Jaylen, my grandson, who always asked, "How are you feeling Nana?" I love you.

Jean and Christine, my two remaining sisters; my brothers, nephews, nieces, cousins and extended family – Much love.

The Baity and Sandor family, who never waiver in their love and support.

Maria, who encouraged me to start journaling –
I appreciate you. A special thanks and much
appreciation for your love, encouragement and
support;

And, to my Heavenly Father, who alone is my
Strength, my Provider and my Healer, I dedicate
"Side-Swiped, My Journey with Peritoneal Cancer;
When the Unexpected Happens" to You.

Especially for

_____

From

_____

Date

_____

Acknowledgments

I cannot find words ample enough to express my appreciation to those who have inspired me along the way and who took time to read the manuscript of this book and give their feedback. The tried and true words "thank you" are inadequate. So, I say accept my special appreciation and gratitude. Of the many who have either been an inspiration or have given of their time, energy and/or efforts to assure the completion of this project.

Those who reviewed the manuscript: Judith Baity for her editorial input and positive energy; Christine Thompson for her helpful comments; Uton Bright who stayed up all night to read and edit the manuscript – I appreciate your loyalty; Pastor D.O. Spence, who came out of retirement to read and edit the manuscript – Thanks for never stop praying for me; Dr. Bertram Melbourne who in his busyness as Professor, Pastor and author, took time to read and edit the manuscript; you never lost your patience when I so many times asked, "Are you through reading?" I appreciate you so much for the wisdom and insight you shared.

Much appreciation and thanks to Danece Goble, my editor, for editing this book and for her personal note of inspiration and encouragement.

I am truly indebted to everyone for their love and support. Yet, beyond and above all else is my gratitude to my God whose unfading love inspires me; whose renewed grace every morning motivates me; whose unending faithfulness is immeasurable, and through whose blessings and touch, this story became a reality. Thank you, Jesus!

Dear Readers,

I refer to myself as a late bloomer in the writing arena. Timing is everything and, nothing happens before the time.

When the unexpected happens, the Lord provides for us, his children. And, so, because of the Lord's guidance and providential leading, "Side-Swiped; My Journey with Peritoneal Cancer; When The Unexpected Happens" was birthed.

I wrote this inspirational book for you. Perhaps you have lost a loved one, or someone is going through cancer or other diseases; a family member or friend is experiencing an illness or hardship. This book will encourage, inspire and give you hope. God is good; God is great; Miracles still happen. Please join me on this journey!

"Now unto him that is able to do exceeding abundantly above all that we ask or think,

according to the power that worketh in us, unto him be glory." Ephesians 3:20-21.

Thank you for your support.

Blessings,

Nora

Table of Contents

Introduction 14

   The Green Light 14

Part I 19

   Knocked Down - A New York State of Mind -
   Christmas 2009 19

   The New Year 2010 21

   I Know My Body 23

   Gastroenterologist (GI) Intervention 26

Part II 30

   The Journey of Faith - OB/GYN Findings 30

   Plan of Action 36

   Oncologist Visit 38

   Prayer Changes Things 40

   Day of Surgery 41

   Post-Surgery and In my Room 45

   April 7th - The Morning After - A Tsunami
   Experience 46

   On My Way Home...50

Education In-Service 56

Post-Op Visit – New Revelation 60

Peritoneal Cancer..61

More Doctor's Visit 65

First Treatment (May 7th)...............................68

In Between Treatment: Back to Work 76

Second Treatment (May 28th) 77

In Between Treatments: Nora Has Left The
Building 83

Desperate Means called for Desperate Measures:
Miracle One 90

What Do I Do Now? My Ad 91

Third Treatment (June 18th): Miracle Two 93

In Between Treatments 95

Wig Happy..97

Acts of Kindness..99

My Two Sons..106

Fourth Treatment (July 9th)...........................110

In Between Treatments....................................111

Fifth Treatment (July 30th)............................113

Sixth Treatment (August 20th) and Reflections
....118

August 30th – Doctor's Appointment 121

September 13th (Day of CT Scan) and My
Mortality 122

Got Hair? 126

September 15th (Visit with Oncologist): Miracle
Three 128

Part III 130

Still Standing - Holy Ground Experience 130

Jaylen is in The House....................................133

Surprise Package 135

When the Unexpected Happens – Can We Talk?
....137

Save for a Rainy Day 144

My Health...145

My Inner Circle 150

Full Circle...152

Close Encounter with the Bible......................154

Songs of Inspiration 157

Sour Sop Fruit 158

Be Careful How We Treat Others...................159

Fruits of the Spirit 161

My Faith Journey 163

Renewed Commitment 171

A Love Connection with Nora 174

Prayers of Thanksgiving and Supplication
Conversations with My Father 176

Thy will be done - Dear Heavenly Father 181

Definitions 182

Introduction

The Green Light

My friend Maria encouraged me to start journaling my experience with cancer, and tell of God's providential leading along the way. She thought putting my words in writing could one day be a blessing to others. I prayerfully sought God's guidance about writing that night.

Since my diagnosis with cancer, my perspective and way of thinking has changed significantly. Previously, I would make decisions on my own without guidance from the Lord, and would just make a big mess of things - nothing seemed to work successfully. I have learned some lessons along the way. Since my diagnosis I made a vow that I would never do anything on my own without asking for guidance from the Lord.

That Friday night, I did not sleep much. My mind was so overwhelmed with the idea of writing an inspirational book of my journey with cancer.

Morning came and I found myself having loud conversations with the Lord, asking Him to show me a sign, to give me some kind of indication that I should undertake this project.

It was Saturday morning and I was getting ready for church. Usually I have an idea of what I wanted to wear to church from the night before. I failed to do that on Friday night. I was still in my bedroom talking to the Lord asking for a sign – something which would be an indication of his approval for me to write an inspirational book of my journey with cancer.

I opened my closet door as I continued talking to the Lord. I told him how he is my father and I am his daughter and how he healed me and made a way out of no way with my hospital bills. "Lord show me something!" I said.

About a year ago, I changed the fluorescent bulbs in my two closets. One worked perfectly all year, I would turn the switch on and the light would come on.

The light in the other closet would not come on when I turned the switch. There would only be a dim flicker of light in the far left corner of the bulb. I would use a fan duster to nudge it gently. The light may or may not come on. I just did not understand why it did not work properly. So, I just left it there and never worried too much about whether or not to have it replaced or to have an electrician check on the problem. This was not on the top of my list.

That morning I turned on the light switch like I usually do and the light came on. I smiled! I said aloud, "Lord is this Your way of telling me that You are giving me the GREEN LIGHT to write this book?" I said again aloud, "Lord, I want to make sure that I am getting Your approval, so I am going to turn off the light, I am going to step out of the closet and come back in. If this is You, let the light come on again when I turn on the light switch." I did exactly that and the light came on.

This may be corny to you, but, to me that was a sign for me to go ahead. In other words, I got the GREEN LIGHT from the Lord. When I got the GREEN LIGHT from the Lord, my heart was filled with joy.

"Side-Swiped, My Journey with Peritoneal Cancer; When The Unexpected Happens" was birthed! It was a day of thanksgiving and praise.

That night I was unable to sleep, not because of the excitement - but because my mind was flooded with the words for this story. If I did not start writing right away, I felt as if I would lose my mind. At 2:00 A.M. I began to write my story and continued writing until 7:00 A.M. that morning. I continued with this same pattern until the book was completed.

Part I

Knocked Down - A New York State of Mind -

Christmas 2009

It is a good thing to rest the mind and body from time to time, to have fun and be happy! Proverbs 17:22 says, *"A merry heart doeth good like a medicine; but a broken spirit drieth the bones."*

For two years, Winston, my oldest son has been promising to bring Jaylen, my grandson for a visit. Winston has sort of exhausted his promises, so I decided to visit them for Christmas in NY. It was October and Christmas was approaching fast; it seemed as if the whole year got condensed into six months! I bought my ticket and I was in a New

York State of Mind. Jason, my youngest son would not be able to make the trip.

December came quickly and it was Christmas! This was very special this year! I was excited to spend some time with my family in New York, especially Jaylen, my grandson. I arrived in New York and was welcomed with twelve inches of snow. It was cold! However, I was used to snow because I lived in New York for twenty-nine years before relocating to North Carolina. My attitude towards the snow and cold was as the young people say, "Whatever!"

My sister Christine and her family drove in from Connecticut to spend time with me. My niece, Marcia had prepared a nice spread of scrumptious foods and desserts. I am not sure how long she spent in the kitchen; but, she has great culinary skills. I was impressed and very proud of her. She made all kinds of things, there was something for the vegan, the vegetarian, and, for those who were not a vegan or a vegetarian. It was a feast! I tasted a little bit of everything and was overstuffed.   It was the holidays, so I had no regrets enjoying the foods that I had not eaten in years.

My visit went by very quickly. Why is it that time passes so swiftly when you are on vacation? The time spent with my family was awesome. My piano selections at the Christmas concert went very well. Mission accomplished! I was on my way back to North Carolina.

The New Year 2010

It was New Year's Eve, and I took the day-off to clean my house, as I did every year. There is a

Caribbean saying, "the cleaner the house when New Year's Eve arrives; the lesser the worries, the lesser the problems for the New Year!" I am not sure I believe it anymore.

I like to stay home on New Year's Eve and New Year's Day, But this year I did not do my usual checklist of resolutions for 2010. Instead, I was very prayerful and it was a time of thanksgiving. I was thankful for my health and that I had lived to see another year. It was 2010 and I was grateful.

While in New York, I did not exactly follow my diet and I did not drink enough water. While I was there my son Winston surrendered his bedroom to me. He wanted me to luxuriate and be comfortable. Usually at night time, I have frequent bathroom visits due to diabetes. So as not to disturb my son during the night, I reduced my water portions significantly. I started to have bladder problems while in New York and even at the airport.

I Know My Body

I always paid attention to my body and knew when something was wrong. Since I know my body so well, I knew that I had a urinary tract infection. In January 2010, I scheduled an appointment with my physician. I will call her Dr. I.M. I went to Dr I.M. and I was right with the diagnosis. I was placed on medication. I did beat up myself a bit for being careless and for not drinking enough water, but I learned my lesson!

Within two weeks of completing the medication, I started to experience unusual cramps in my abdomen. They were very mild, but noticeable. I made a mental note of the cramps and decided to monitor them!

The cramps became severe over the next couple of days. I thought to myself, "What in the world is going on?" "What did I eat?" I blamed myself big time for going off my diet in New York. As time went on the cramps continued. They felt like slight labor pains, at times I had to hold on to something and take brief breaths as if I was in labor.

Again, I knew my body very well and this was not normal. I scheduled another visit to Dr. I.M. The diagnosis was Helicobacter pylori also called H. Pylori (the bacteria responsible for most ulcers and many cases of stomach inflammation). I thought to myself, "How did this happen?" I know that when I eat certain foods that I have not eaten in a while, my stomach may or may not tolerate those foods – but H. Pylori?

I was placed on medication and took eight antibiotics a day for two weeks. I noticed that the side effects of the medication were the same as my symptoms. The pain was so unbearable that I cried! I did not know that I had such a strong tolerance for pain until this experience. On a scale of 0-10, the pain was at 9 and that is no exaggeration!

Listen to your body!

Pay attention to what it is telling you!

Know your body!

Do not play the "wait and see" game with the symptoms that you have. Do not procrastinate with your health. Seek medical consultation immediately. Do not be afraid or intimidated to inform your physician of any symptoms that are unusual. Be aggressive with your physician, it is your body and your health.

Gastroenterologist (GI) Intervention

I completed the medication and there was no relief. It seemed as if the cramping found its way to my rectum. The pain made me feel like I constantly needed to go to the bathroom. I had never experienced such unusual pain before. It was terrible and unbearable. I knew that something was wrong. I was on a mission to find out what was wrong with my body.

I decided I need to take things into my own hands.

In February, I scheduled an appointment with my Gastroenterologist, who I will call, Dr. G.I. I was not afraid of a colonoscopy; it was the bowel preparation that I did not like. You, know, the combination of the powdered mixture along with one gallon of a juice, which results in a horrible tasting drink. Yes, the drink that will make your body shudder, shiver and cause chill bumps to find their way to the surface of your arms!

It is best to follow the instructions, so that the colon area is nice and clear. The thought of cheating and not drinking all of the mixture and having another colonoscopy scheduled was not an option for me.

The colonoscopy was scheduled and done immediately. Dr. G.I. found some polyps, which were removed and biopsied. They were benign. I was grateful the colonoscopy was done   Praise God!

Dr. G.I. was aware of the H. Pylori diagnosis, she recommended that I take an *Align* Probiotic supplement. *Align* is a probiotic that naturally replenishes the digestive system with healthy bacteria. Probiotics are good bacteria essential for many vital body functions, including healthy digestion.

I was grateful and thankful for the results of the colonoscopy, however, the cramping continued. Dr. G.I. called to follow up on my progress. She was made aware that there was no change. She said, "Nora, this has been going on too long, I am going to schedule you for a CT Scan." The appointment was made for the CT Scan immediately.

A CT Scan is a scan that uses a computer linked to an X-ray machine which produces detailed pictures of the inside of the body.

The CT Scan was done in March. It revealed that in the abdomen there was a small amount of intra-peritoneal fluid seen in the right peri-pelvic space and along the paracolic gutters bilaterally, and that there was fluid in the small bowel mesentery. Soft tissue stranding was seen within the omental fat and to a lesser degree the mesenteric fat. Similar findings were also identified in the pelvis with strandings. There was a small left renal cyst and tiny gallstones in the dependent portion of the gallbladder. I was suspicious and concerned with the results. What does all of the above mean? None of this looked good!

Dr. G.I. referred me to an Obstetrician and Gynecologist (OB/GYN) very quickly.

Part II

The Journey of Faith - OB/GYN Findings

One week later, I was in the office of an OB/GYN for consultation. I will call her, Dr. O.G. A vaginal ultrasound was done. This procedure involves using a probe to obtain close contact images of the uterus and ovaries.

The procedure took 30 minutes; however, it seemed forever. I was escorted to Dr. O.G's office for the results of the ultrasound. She stepped away from behind her desk and sat next to me to discuss the findings. Even if the news would be grim, sitting next to me helped to put me at ease. After what seemed like hours of discussion, her comment was, "I know that the information must be overwhelming." My response was, "I am a big girl, and I can handle it." My response was not "cocky" nor was it "full of myself," it was confidence; it was my will to fight. I was ready to fight - I was not about to be knocked down or out!

I was told that my right ovary was larger than the usual size. Each ovary is the size of an almond. There was also a shadow around the area of the ovary. The images confirmed the results of the CT Scan. Blood was drawn to run a CA-125 which would determine if there was cancer.

The CA-125 is a blood test used to measure the level of CA-125, a tumor marker that is often found in higher-than-normal amounts in the blood of women with ovarian or peritoneal cancer.

The laboratory results of the CA-125 indicated that the number was beyond the range for "normal". It therefore indicated that I had ovarian cancer.

I was told that surgery had to be done possibly a full hysterectomy. Surgery was inevitable and an Oncologist would perform it. For me, the decision was a no brainer, I agreed for the surgery to be done. I was way beyond childbearing years and those female organs had fulfilled their potential. Surgery was scheduled to be done on April 6, 2010.

I was offered the option of robotic surgery or traditional surgery. Information was provided on robotic surgery, which benefits both the physician and the patient. It reduces blood loss; it is less invasive; it shortens hospital stay and recovery times. The robotic surgery would not be performed in the town where I lived. I, therefore, opted for the traditional surgery.

I was relieved that the CT Scan and the CA-125 revealed what was wrong with me. I could now concentrate on how to beat cancer. I was not ready to die. My prayer was, "Lord, please handpick the physician(s) who will provide my medical care. Give them wisdom, knowledge and understanding."

After all of the information was presented to me, I got in my car. My mind was overwhelmed with questions. I had conversations with myself on my ride home.

"Why was I not angry?"

"Where were my tears?"

"Why was I not crying?"

"Did I accept the news?"

"Was I in denial?"

"Did I have any emotions?"

"Was something wrong with me?"

There were no tears and no anger, I accepted the diagnosis. The emotions I had were positive not negative. I knew that negative emotions would have produced negative outcomes, such as fear and anxiety. I would have become a worrywart! The negative emotions would have adversely affected my health and hindered my wellness.

I was not in denial and I did not question the Lord or challenge His faithfulness. I knew that I trusted and served a God who was and is still in the healing business. I had faith that He was not going to leave or forsake me. I prayed to the Lord to cover me and give me strength to endure the trials ahead of me.

As far as I knew cancer had never been in my families medical history. Annual pap smears were done on time and the results were always normal. Annual mammograms were done and there were no abnormalities. I was diligent and kept up with annual medical related appointments. For the first time in my life, cancer, a dreaded disease would now be part of my family medical history.

Sometimes our path is crooked or a "zig-zag." Our path may not always be straight. At the end of the path, there could be new revelations that could begin a new journey. Mine was a journey of health issues. Had I not visited New York, who is to say how long it would have taken for me to discover that I had cancer? Perhaps, it would have been too late for me, perhaps, there would have been no hope.

Each health issue led me closer to what was going on in my body. The diagnosis of a Urinary Tract Infection led to the diagnosis of H. Pylori which led to a colonoscopy. This procedure led to a CT Scan, which led to a vaginal ultrasound and CA-125. The crooked path led me to the diagnosis of cancer, a disease that could potentially kill me.

In my alone time, the title of a song came to mind that says; *My Soul Is Anchored In The Lord*. The words of this song spoke to the "storms" I was experiencing in my life. Nevertheless, I was comforted and reassured that regardless of the diagnosis of cancer, my soul is anchored in the Lord.

Plan of Action

I switched into mission mode and developed a check list of things to do prior to my surgery. I had conversations with my two sons about the surgery and the reasons for it. Their reactions were like night and day. The youngest, Jason was calm and prayerful. I believe he was scared. But, he did not show it. My oldest, Winston, lost it. This was a natural reaction and I understood it. The news of my illness was difficult for both of them. Other than a cold or an occasional flu, they have never seen me sick. I asked that they both be strong, trust and have faith in God.

I also needed to update my two sisters, Jean and Christine. I called Jean immediately to let her know about the surgery. She was about to leave on vacation to the Caribbean and would not be back for a while. My sister Christine committed to come and stay with me for one week following my discharge from the hospital. I had conversations with some other family members and friends about the surgery. I did not go into details because I did not want to overwhelm them with too much information.

I advised the appropriate personnel at work regarding the surgery. FMLA (Family Medical

Leave Act) was requested and approved. I would have to return to work in six to twelve weeks.

I made an appointment with my hair stylist to have my hair French-braided. During my hospital stay, I did not want to worry about maintaining it.

Oncologist Visit

I had an appointment to meet with the Oncologist prior to my surgery. I will call the Oncologist, Dr. O.N.C. For this appointment I had to go to the Cancer Center for the first time. I was not mentally or emotionally prepared for this experience.

When I arrived everywhere I looked I saw were sick people. Some were in wheel-chairs, others used canes, some had oxygen tanks and surgical masks that covered their nose. Each patient had a hand-held device that lit up and buzzed when it was time to go to the lab to have blood drawn, or to the treatment area for chemotherapy. I could see the effect that cancer had on these patients, especially the older ones.

I thought, Lord, help me and have mercy on me! It was overwhelming and my blood pressure became elevated.

A physical exam was done and I was provided with information about the surgery. Preliminary tests and admission paperwork were completed for the surgery. Despite having already done a colonoscopy, it was recommended that a bowel preparation be done the night before the surgery. "Here we go again," I thought! I would have to drink the horrible mixture again. My mind was made up and I would do what I had to do.

Prayer Changes Things

I went to church that Saturday, April 3rd and asked for prayer from my church family. In times of uncertainty, dilemma, and catastrophic circumstances, I called upon the Prayer Warriors. I had friends and family all over the country that interceded for me 24/7 during my journey with cancer.

Matthew 18:20 says, *"For where two or three are gathered together in my name, there am I in the midst of them."*

Isaiah 53:5 says, *"That with his stripes, that we are healed."*

I was claiming healing from the inside out!

I was raised with the notion to always pray. As a little girl, a popular prayer was, *"Gentle Jesus, meek and mild, look upon a little child..."* When I was still very young, I memorized the Lord's Prayer and the 23rd Psalm. Years later, my prayers became personal, they became my own words and my own petition to the Lord.

Prayer is my life-line with a direct connection to the Lord. It is a telephone with unlimited lines. There are no monthly installments and it is free of charge. I have been talking to the Lord for a long time and I have tapped into those lines frequently. What a privilege and what awesome accessibility we have.

Day of Surgery

It was April 6th. I was scheduled to arrive at the hospital at 8:00 A.M. I woke up early and was at peace.

When I turned 50, one of my requests to the Lord was that He would grant me peace going forward in all of my trials and tribulations.

Colossians 3:15 says, *"Let the peace of God rule in your hearts."* The American Heritage College dictionary, third edition, defines *rule* as "the governing power or its possession or use; or authority." I wanted the peace of God to have authority or power in my heart.

My son, Jason, a full-time student, dropped me off at the hospital that morning. He planned to return later that day after his classes. I did not want Jason to miss classes, so I encouraged him to attend classes and come to the hospital later. I know that was difficult for him to do. Before he left, he held my hands and prayed for the Lord to be with me, and to guide the hands of the physicians. He also prayed for a quick recovery. It was a powerful and meaningful prayer of faith. That was an emotional moment for both of us.

Miranda, a close friend of mine arrived shortly after I did. I remember she held my hands and said, "I want you to know that I will be here for you all day." I was so appreciative and blessed by her presence. We sat in silence most of the time. We were lost in our own private thoughts.

We were escorted to a room where I would be prepped for surgery. Miranda sat next to the bed where I laid. The "prep nurse" arrived and went through the preliminaries. As my gown was partially removed, Miranda very swiftly (like lightning) spun around and faced the wall so that I could have privacy. I burst into a laugh at her wonder-woman stunt. Miranda did not get up, she remained scated and in a swift like manner spun the chair around. It's as if she had rehearsed this drill or had done it before and knew what to do. We laughed together, we hugged, and said our "see you later" and "I love you" pleasantries. I was ready to be wheeled to the waiting area in the surgery suite.

The Oncologist and the Anesthesiologist reassured me that I was in good hands. My OB/GYN physician would assist the Oncologist with surgery. Incidentally, the Oncologist who performed my surgery was not the physician who was scheduled initially. I was not surprised by the change since there was a group of Oncology physicians who alternated as needed.

I prayed quietly, knowing that the Lord knew all things and I was not worried.

As I was wheeled into the operating room, I continued to pray silently. As the anesthesia was administered I silently prayed the 23rd Psalm until my body succumbed to the anesthesia:

"The Lord is my shepherd; I shall not want. He maketh me to lie down in green pastures: He leadeth me beside the still waters. He restoreth

my soul: he leadeth me in the paths of righteousness for his name's sake, Yea, though I walk through the valley of the shadow of death, I will fear no evil: for thou art with me; thy rod and thy staff they comfort me. Thou preparest a table before me in the presence of mine enemies; thou anointest my head with oil; my cup runneth over. Surely goodness and mercy shall follow me all the days of my life: and I will dwell in the house of the Lord forever."

Post-Surgery and In my Room

Hours later, I was in my room, not too cognizant of who was in the room or what was said. Still under anesthesia, the images around me were blurred. Subconsciously, I hoped that my closest friends and Jason were there. Still under anesthesia and pain medication I was not doing a lot of talking and was in and out of reality. I thought I heard that the surgery was successful, a partial hysterectomy was done. A biopsy of the ovaries revealed cancer and my appendix was also removed. I have type 2-diabetes and was unable to take metformin prior to and after my surgery. During the night, I was given insulin periodically so I did not get much sleep.

I was aware that another friend of mine spent the night. I remembered that she massaged my feet when they were cold. I truly appreciated that.

April 7th - The Morning After - A Tsunami Experience

Morning came and I was in pain. I was not sure what I heard after the surgery, so I wanted my physicians to update me on the surgery. I was told that some of my female organs and appendix were re-sectioned, other parts excised.

It was confirmed that I had ovarian cancer which would require chemotherapy. Apparently my abdomen was a big mess due to cancer! I felt as if I was having a Tsunami experience on dry land! I remember thinking that I was Side-Swiped and the journey ahead of me had begun.

I know that after the vaginal ultrasound was done, there was a possibility that there could be cancer. On the other hand, optimism had kicked in and just maybe, there would be no cancer. I was still not angry; there were still no tears. I accepted the diagnosis.

I prayed silently,

"I lift up my eyes unto the hills from whence cometh my help. My help cometh from the Lord

which made the heaven and earth. He will not suffer thy foot to be moved: he that keepeth thee will not slumber, Behold, he that keepeth Israel shall neither slumber nor sleep. The Lord is thy keeper: the Lord is thy shade upon thy right hand. The sun shall not smite thee by day, nor the moon by night. The Lord shall preserve thee from all evil: he shall preserve thy soul. The Lord shall preserve thy going out and thy coming in from this time forth, and even for evermore."

Psalms 121 would become one of my daily prayers and my spiritual anthem. I personalized it and changed the words "thy" to "my" and "thee" to "me."

The day after surgery I was given instructions to get out of bed and do some walking. I was obedient, however, it was so difficult to walk. Just getting out of bed was very painful.

Bathroom visits were frequent for me during the night. On each side of the bed, there were handrails to prevent me from falling out of bed. They were a hindrance when bathroom visits were necessary. I was unable to get out of bed with any speed; it was a struggle which led to embarrassing moments before I made it to the bathroom. Did I use the call bell? Yes. Let's say, things do happen – I was helpless and embarrassed.

As an independent person, two of my biggest concerns were the fear of being helpless and that of having to depend on someone to do things for me. I had a close encounter with the fear of helplessness after my surgery.

My pride did not prevent the negotiation for a bed-pan. It was inevitable! My hospital stay lasted for four days. My time there was painful and depressing due to my fear of helplessness.

I had a visit from the Community Services leader from my church. Her son, a pastor was with her. He held my hands and prayed with me. I needed that! She and other members of the Tuesday mornings study group sent me get well cards from time to time.

My church family knew that I had surgery, but I made the decision to keep my diagnosis private. It was a personal thing for me.

The days of recovery went by slowly. Jason and close friends came and went. Finally I was discharged with instructions on Friday, April 9th. Jason was on time and I was going home.

On My Way Home

On the ride home, I asked Jason what were his emotions and thoughts on the day of my surgery as he left the hospital parking lot? He said, "Mom, the surgery was out of my control, why worry? I turned everything over to God in whom I trust. I had faith that the surgery would be successful." There was silence for the duration of the trip home.

Home is where the heart is. Be it ever so humble there is no place like home. I was home, in my own bed and familiar surroundings. I was grateful and thankful that my life was spared. I was alive! Thank you Lord!

I always was a slim person. Between April 6th and the 9th, I had already lost eight pounds. When I looked at my legs, the skin was already sagging. I was troubled but I kept that information to myself.

I was once told if I ever became seriously ill, my weight loss would quickly show because I would be very thin. Major surgery took a toll on my slim frame.

While still in the hospital I was given food, but I had no appetite. I did not eat much of the food, those four days, which also contributed to my weight loss. I just do not like hospital food.

When I arrived home I made a phone call to a dear friend of mine who I grew up with. She had breast cancer in 2009 and was now a cancer survivor. She was very helpful and empathetic. I knew that she would know exactly what I was going through. There is an expression "You would not wish this or that on your worst enemy!" Well, if we did have any enemies we would not wish cancer on them much less anyone else. It's a dreadful disease!

From time to time my friend would call and pray with me, she would even sing to me on the phone. Her encouragement helped me tremendously.

I called Marcia, my niece and updated her on the results of the surgery. It was important to let her know, since she would be the liaison to my sister, Jean and other family members.

On the evening of April 9th, my sister Christine arrived. I was grateful that she came and relieved that Jason would not be too overwhelmed with my illness. That Saturday, my friends and their family visited and they provided lunch for us.

The menu: Lasagna and Okra – compliments of the Baity and the Sandor family. The Okra was for me. The slimy texture did not bother me, my focus was on the benefits of it. Okra is chock full of vitamins. It prevents constipation and is an excellent laxative. Okra worked for me and was part of my diet after surgery and during chemotherapy.

That day there was a lot of laughter, even though I could not do much of it due to my discomfort. It was so good to see them.

I was so blessed that my younger sister found the time to visit me and to take care of me. She pampered me and cooked all of my meals. My appetite was slowly coming back. She juiced fresh organic carrots, beets, celery and apples daily for me.

My sister loves the outdoors. She pulled weeds and planted the perennials I received from well wishers. I would sit outside and get some sun while she transplanted flowers and plants in the yard.

My stomach muscles were still extremely sore. The skin on the left side of my stomach was numb. I could barely feel anything on that side. The incision was vertically done so that it would enable the doctors to view the entire abdominal area and the "stage" of the cancer. This meant there would be more muscle to cut through, which contributed to the numbness in my skin.

For eight weeks, I had to get accustomed to sleeping on my back. I missed sleeping on my side and on my stomach. There were some nights that I would turn on my side inadvertently and I would moan and groan in pain. It took much effort to get out of bed, and even greater effort to walk. I had no idea that I used my stomach muscles so much just to get out of bed. It was a really uncomfortable process. I developed a technique on how to get out of bed and walk around the house. I would lay very close to the edge of the bed flat on my back, supporting my body on my elbows; I would then scoot up close to the headboard; hold on to the headboard, and slowly swing both legs to the edge of the bed unto the floor.

Just thinking about the technique still makes me feel tired. Yet, it was less painful than getting out of bed the traditional way. More importantly, it worked for me.

Walking was another matter! I would support my tummy with both hands; crouch my body a bit, and then dragging my feet, I made tiny annoying steps around the house.

Education In-Service

My sister and I attended an educational session at the Cancer Center regarding chemotherapy. We agreed that it would be best for her to attend so she could better understand and learn about cancer and how to be most effective in assisting me. A wealth of information was provided.

The facilitators told us that Chemotherapy (also called chemo) is a type of cancer treatment that uses drugs to destroy cancer cells. The same drug that destroys cancer cells also destroys the good cells. This included cells that line the mouth and intestines, cells in the bone marrow that make blood cells, and cells that make the hair grow. Chemotherapy causes side effects when it harms these healthy cells.

The doctor decides which chemotherapy drugs to use based upon the type of cancer one has. Other health problems are also taken into consideration, i.e. diabetes or heart disease, etc. I am a diabetic.

Chemotherapy is given in cycles. This means that chemotherapy treatment is followed by a period of rest. The rest period gives the body a chance to build new healthy cells. Chemotherapy may be given by injection, intra-arterial, intraperitoneal, intravenous, topically or orally. In my case, it was given intravenously, meaning it would go directly into a vein.

Some of the side effects of chemotherapy include: fatigue, hair loss, and nausea, loss of appetite, vomiting, diarrhea, constipation, sores in the mouth, decreased blood cell counts and infection. Each person's experience with chemotherapy is different. The doctors recommended that I avoid crowded areas, such as restaurants, super markets, and potluck events to prevent infections.

During chemo it is extremely important to stay hydrated. Water, ice chips, fruit juices, soups, broth, decaffeinated teas, and popsicles were all recommended to prevent dehydration.

The information for chemotherapy was very overwhelming for both my sister and I.

Before I began my chemo treatment I decided to get an extremely short haircut, so I would not be too traumatized with the loss of my hair. I jokingly told my sister not to get any ideas about her cutting my hair. Soon it was time for my sister to leave and return to her home in Connecticut. I dreaded that day!

I have worked in the healthcare industry for about 26 years in administrative positions. I have read a lot of health related articles. While nothing read matches the reality of the situation, the truth of the matter is that I have never read any information on cancer. It did not even cross my mind. Diagnosed with cancer I was forced to speed read everything that I could find on the disease that had found itself in my body.

I know that God did not give me a spirit of fear; therefore, either I was going to be fearful and let cancer overwhelm me, succumbed to the disease and die from it or I could believe that there was nothing too hard for the Lord. I decided on the latter, and prayed for healing.

Post-Op Visit – New Revelation

My post op appointment was on April 20th. It was about two weeks after my surgery. Dr. O.N.C. the Oncologist said the incision was healing nicely. I was told that a separate consultation with a pathologist confirmed that I had peritoneal cancer. My case represented a diagnostic challenge due to the morphology not being as simple as in the usual case of peritoneal serous carcinoma. There was concern about the fluid in my abdomen as well as its origin. Dr. O.N.C. opened the possibility of the need for more surgery.

Have you ever heard the phrase, "the devil is a liar?" Well, that was what I said to myself as I was told there may be more surgery.

Other problems in my abdomen remained untouched or left alone for fear that I would need a colostomy.

What does all of this mean? That the cancer was all over my abdomen and it was serious.

I did not want to worry my family about the seriousness of the cancer. It would have been too much for them. I kept it to myself and was calm with the new revelation of a new diagnosis. Why worry? My focus was not on negative emotions. I was focused on healing!

Peritoneal Cancer

I did some research on WebMD since I had never heard of this type of cancer.

Peritoneal Cancer is a rare cancer. It develops in a thin layer of tissue that lines the abdomen. It also covers the uterus, bladder and rectum. Made of epithelial cells, this structure is called the peritoneum. It produces a fluid that helps organs move smoothly inside the abdomen. Peritoneal Cancer starts in the peritoneum. So it is called peritoneal cancer. Peritoneum cancer acts and looks like ovarian cancer. Mainly because the surface of the ovaries is made up of epithelial cells, as is the peritoneum. Therefore, peritoneum cancer and a type of ovarian cancer cause similar symptoms.

Peritoneum cancer can occur anywhere in the abdominal space. It affects the surface of the organs contained in the peritoneum. WebMD says that the causes of peritoneal cancer are unknown and there are different theories about how it begins.

Some believe it comes from ovarian tissue implants left in the abdomen during fetal development. Others think the peritoneum undergoes a change that makes it more like the ovaries.

Older age is one of the risks factor for peritoneal cancer. Just as with ovarian cancer, peritoneal cancer can be hard to detect in the early stages. The symptoms are vague and hard to pinpoint. When clear symptoms do occur, the disease has often progressed. The symptoms resemble those of ovarian cancer. Many of these symptoms are due to a buildup of fluid in the abdomen.

Symptoms of peritoneal cancer may include:

- Feeling of fullness, even after a light meal;

- Abdominal discomfort or pain from gas, indigestion;

- pressure, swelling, bloating or cramps;

- Nausea or diarrhea;

- Constipation;

- Frequent urination;

- Loss of appetite;

- Unexplained weight gain or loss;

- Abnormal vaginal bleeding;

After I read this information I thought that this type of cancer I had was sneaky and rare. I also realized that peritoneal cancer was not necessarily a family history disease, based upon the different theories as to how it begins.

Hi, my name is Nora, and I have peritoneal cancer!

More Doctor's Visit

I was scheduled to meet with another physician on May 3rd. I will call her Dr. M.O. This physician monitored my progress and requested labs to be done frequently in the month of May. Prior to check-ups each month, labs were done. Dr. M.O. would look at the results of the white and red blood cells and platelets, etc.

Different prescriptions were written for me to take prior to each treatment and for nausea symptoms. At each exam Dr. M.O. asked me questions about each side effect, to determine how chemotherapy affected me. Did I experience any appetite changes, any constipation, diarrhea, fatigue, mouth sores, skin and nail changes?

The drugs used for chemotherapy and the pain medication caused constipation, so I made sure that my diet consisted of whole grains, oatmeal, dried beans, fresh fruits and water.

What impressed me was that I was always asked by Dr. M.O. whether or not I needed to talk to someone about what I was going through. While I did not require that particular service, I was pleased that the service was available. I was told that doctors and nurses were on call 24/7 for any questions.

I was so impressed with Dr. M.O's professionalism and the patient/doctor relationship I had with her. She was so soft-spoken; her voice had a calming effect on me. A great doctor!

My first treatment was scheduled on May 7th and thereafter every three weeks. I was also told by Dr. M.O. that after each treatment an injection would be administered, depending on my white and red blood cell count.

Since chemotherapy decreases the number of the white blood cells, it was important to avoid infections. Some types of chemotherapy make it harder for bone marrow to produce new white blood cells. White blood cells help the body fight infections. Injections would be administered when recommended by the physician.

Extra precautions and much care had to be taken when undergoing chemotherapy. If a fever is 100.5 or higher, the physician must know immediately. I monitored my temperature very frequently. Hand washing with soap and water was very important using the 20 seconds time frame required.

First Treatment (May 7th)

My treatments were scheduled for Fridays. In preparation for my first chemotherapy, I was prescribed Dexamethasone and took the night before each chemotherapy. Dexamethasone is in a class of drugs called steroids. The drug prevents the release of substances in the body that causes inflammation. There were ten pills (five were taken twelve hours before my 9:00 A.M. appointment and the other five were taken six hours before). This meant that I had to get up at 3:00 A.M. in the morning to take the last five doses. Each dose was taken with food. I was restless that night and did not get much sleep. I was fearful that I would sleep beyond 3:00 A.M.

The first time I took the pills, I had a hard time swallowing them, because they were so many to take at one time. The pills were bitter! The taste lingered in my mouth for a while.

Jason dropped me off for my first treatment. He held my hands and prayed with me. It was another emotional moment for the two of us.

This was my first chemotherapy. I did not know what to expect. I had embarked on a journey that caused me to have a bit of anxiety and fear. It was the fear of the unknown. As I entered the waiting area, I felt like a little girl who was lost and was not sure where I was going and what I would discover.

Admission paperwork for outpatient procedure was done. I was given the hand-held device that would light up. It buzzed when it was time for labs and chemotherapy. Labs were done first, then, I was escorted to the treatment area.

My steps were very slow as I entered the treatment area. I held on tightly to my pocket book, lunch bag and book. I took in the surroundings that would be my home on an outpatient basis for several months.

I was greeted and paired up with a Nurse who would administer the drugs Taxol and Carboplatin through an IV and into my vein. The nurse would supervise my treatment. Taxol is a cancer medication that interferes with growth of cancer cells and slows their growth in the body.

Taxol can lower blood cells that help the body fight infections. It can make it easier for someone to bleed easier from an injury or get sick from being around others who are ill. The blood will need to be tested on a regular basis to ensure that the blood cells do not get too low.

Taxol is given in a hospital setting or clinic by a nurse or other trained health professional. It is to be given slowly through an IV fusion and can take up to 24 hours to complete. Other drugs may be given to prevent a serious allergic reaction to Taxol. Burning, pain, or swelling around the IV needle must be reported to the nurse.

Emergency medical help is required when there are hives, difficulty breathing; feeling like you might pass out; swelling of the face, lip, tongue, or throat, seizure, fever, chills, body aches, white patches or sores inside the mouth or on the lips, and loss of hair. Taxol can cause other side effects.

Carboplatin treats cancer of the ovaries, lung, head and neck and is used in combination with other medicines. Like Taxol, it is administered in a hospital setting or cancer treatment center by a nurse or other trained professional. It is given through a needle placed in a vein.

Some of the side effects are similar to that of Taxol. It can cause nausea and or vomiting in most people; changes in vision; numbness, tingling, or burning in the hands, feet, arms, legs or feet; ringing in the ears or trouble hearing and like Taxol, hair loss.

My first experience of the administering of the IV did not go very smoothly. My veins are very thin and they did not cooperate, they collapsed. I was in tears! The nurse was allowed two attempts to do the administering of the IV. If unsuccessful, another nurse would take over. Another nurse took over and found the vein successfully. The back of my hands would be the area for administering the IV. I learned that another name for a nurse who administered the IV was called a "sticker."

After an hour or so, the drug/fluid in the IV stopped. I had to go through the IV process again. I cried so much. I had no apologies for my tears. My first experience was not an encouraging one.

Since my veins were thin, I was presented with another option a "Port" for IV chemotherapy. A port is a small, round disc made of plastic or metal that is placed under the skin. A catheter connects the port to a large vein, in the chest area and a nurse insert a needle into the port to give chemotherapy or draw blood. I watched the process on several patients. I was intimidated by it and chose not to use a port.

What was important for me was to find a "sticker" who was skilled at finding a vein without any problems. I got to know a great "sticker" and my process went smoothly thereafter.

My glucose level was escalated due to the medication I took the night before so insulin was administered during chemotherapy. This would continue throughout the duration of my chemotherapy.

The first treatment lasted for about six hours. I was quiet and stayed in my chair except for restroom visits. The volunteers were so wonderful. They asked if I needed a warm blanket, crackers, or soup? I accepted the warm blanket due the cold temperature. God bless them for their volunteer services.

Chemotherapy was administered in an open area. I observed that the other patients slept during the treatments. My body would not let me sleep, my eyes were as bright as a stadium light bulb!

The first treatment ended. I had previously filled prescriptions for nausea with instructions to take in the P.M. and in the A.M. after each treatment. I took the nausea medicines after my first chemotherapy. That was the only time that I took the nausea medicine. My physician, Dr. M.O. was amazed that I was not nauseous throughout the chemotherapy.

My first treatment was over, I could rest over the weekend. The treatments left me with a horrible metal taste in my mouth which lasted for two days. During this time nothing tasted right, even water tasted like it was dirty or stale. This horrible taste continued throughout the treatments.

I used a tongue scraper to clean my tongue. It was recommended that a soft toothbrush was used. To avoid mouth sores, I brushed my teeth with baking soda instead of toothpaste. Baking soda is an ingredient in some brands of toothpaste. I liked baking soda and now alternate with regular toothpaste.

In Between Treatment: Back to Work

I was concerned that chemotherapy would make me look older. It did not! I have never looked my actual age. At the young age of 63, I look more in my mid 50's. For real!! Am I vain? No. The Lord has blessed me with youthfulness. I felt confident returning to work.

Six weeks had gone by. It was time to return to work. I was emotionally, physically and mentally prepared. It was back to the grind stone and I was ready!

My weight loss was evident. Therefore, I was careful of my choice of colors and how I dressed. I wore a black and white summer dress the first day back to work. It was accentuated with red accessories. It was good to see my co-workers. I believe the feeling was mutual.

I notified appropriate personnel of the cancer diagnosis and that chemotherapy had begun. Approval was granted to continue with the previously arranged 32 hour week at work. A portion of my job responsibilities were performed by someone in my absence. She did a wonderful job. It was not difficult to get back in the work mode and to manage it well.

I was concerned about fatigue so I made sure that I did not go beyond eight hours each day. I was blessed to be alive and able to work. I was grateful.

Second Treatment (May 28th)

The usual preparation was done the night before. The pills were still a challenge. I had no choice but to swallow them. At the hospital registration was completed. I got my hand-held device and waited to be buzzed for Labs and the treatment area.

I did not have to be escorted to the treatment area this time. I was now familiar with my surroundings and knew where to go. Anxiety and fear were gone and I was more confident. I was always quiet during the treatments. I would close my eyes or read a book. At times, I made eye contact with other patients and smiled.

I talked with a patient who was next to me. We spoke about our illnesses. She had a bag with some gifts that represented Peace and Tranquility, etc. She gave me two. I shared some thoughts with her. I even pointed out that I prayed for peace on the outcome of my illness and trusted the Lord to heal me. Yet, I was open to God's will and ready to follow God's leading.

The treatment ended and I was scheduled for the first injection which would be in series of three. The injection administered was Neupogen. This medication stimulates the blood system (bone marrow) to make white blood cells, and to help me fight infections. This medication is given to those whose ability to make white blood cells has been reduced. It is given usually once a day until the proper blood counts are reached.

After the series of three injections ended, as I walked in the lobby area, I again saw the woman with whom I had the conversation about our illnesses. She asked, "Are you the woman who sat next to me in the treatment area?" When I responded affirmatively, she shared with me the fact that she had thought about some of the things I had said to her. In fact it meant a lot to her. She further noted that I had in fact inspired her.

I was humbled and excited by her kind words. I saw the need for us to be open to the leading and guidance of the Spirit. Sometimes, we do not know when and how the Lord will use us to bring blessings and inspiration to others. Also, you just do not know what part of a conversation will touch someone's heart or speak to their lives. We therefore need to be open. When she told me that I had inspired her, I saw it as a compliment.

The Web's definition of *inspiration* is the "Arousal of the mind to special unusual activity or creativity; a special influence on the minds of human beings."

I thought about the definition because of a similar experience I had earlier. At my high school reunion in 2007, a former class-mate said, "You have no idea how much you have inspired your peers from your elementary and high school years."

This was news to me since I look back at those days as being that time when we were so young and giddy with no thought of a care. Yes, we did not take life very seriously. Did I set out to inspire someone? No, however, those are the times when we make our greatest impact.

Looking back I saw what may have influenced their thinking. I must admit that I was an attractive young woman. I was popular with the girls and boys. I began playing the piano at a young age. I was a Spelling Bee champion for the Parish of St. James. (A Parish is similar to a "State.") I directed the choir that consisted of many of my peers, and I was a member of our high school trio.

All of these activities placed me in a high profile position. Perhaps it was the accomplishment of these things at a young age that might have inspired someone. If that was the case, I am humbled and I give the praise to the Lord who gave me the talents and directed my young life.

About two weeks after my second treatment, my hair started to fall out in small clumps in the comb. My weight also began to drop; As a result, my clothes began to get very baggy. To address the situation and make it a little more tolerable, if only for me, I began to dress differently. I noted that skirts and dresses did not make me look as slim. I began wearing more skirts and dresses. I also noted that colors that were bright and vibrant did a lot for me, so I began wearing bright and cheerful colors. The trick was that people focused on the bright colors that I wore and not on my slimness.

In Between Treatments: Nora Has Left The Building

June 14th was another regular day at work. A celebration was scheduled to be held that day. The dress code was to wear anything red, white or blue. I did just that.

I had my usual oatmeal for breakfast. I looked at the neatly stacked workload, the in-box and the e-mails. My work day started out in a typical fashion. About mid-morning I was summoned to the office. This was not unusual but what followed was.

On arrival I was told that my position was terminated. While I was not prepared for the news, I tried to be very calm. Whether it was a change of outlook after the diagnosis of cancer or that I was in a state of shock, or it was a combination of these factors; whatever it was, I was definitely Side-Swiped for the second time within two months.

My thoughts began to race. First cancer! Now, my job! What would be next! I did not even remind the bearer of the news that I was recovering from cancer and was on chemotherapy. I did say, however, that I gave the company 110% at all times.

A security guard stood outside my office door as I gathered my few personal belongings. I resented this though I understood it was routine and his duty. It sent a message I did not like.

A co-worker and dear friend, helped packed my stuff. She accompanied me to my car. I appreciated her assistance immensely. Throughout our professional relationship, I have come to love her as an older sister. She loved the Lord and would share a "word from the scriptures" with me all the time.

On the way home I thought that after eleven years of employment with this company, my position had been terminated; I was going through chemotherapy; I now have no medical/dental benefits; I have mortgage responsibilities; I was jobless! This was not timely. It was totally unexpected! I was determined then that I would put my trust in God and would leave the rest to Him.

When I lived in New York, homelessness was seen on the subways and, on the streets. It was everywhere! Here in North Carolina, as I drove to work around 8:00 A.M in the morning, there was a certain area where I would see homeless people with their small bundles, their only possessions perhaps making their way to another spot to pass time until nightfall.

My heart would ache, and I always wondered, what circumstances or situations caused someone to be homeless. What are some of the factors that contribute to homelessness? It is the untimely loss of jobs; inability to provide for the family; hard times and the incapability to keep up with mortgage payments. It felt awful when everything crumbled around me. On the day my position was terminated, I had a full understanding how quickly someone could be a victim of homelessness. I acknowledged that dilemmas, problems, unexpected situations, financial obligations and the loss of a job could combine to make me become homeless. The reality of my situation now loomed large.

Since childhood I had been taught to trust the One who owned the cattle on a thousand hills. This was now my opportunity to put theory into practice. Could I pass the test?

When I got home, I was very angry. I had already accepted the diagnosis of cancer. My focus was to be healed. Now, my income was gone. "Enough is enough!" "Was I "punked?" "Was this a test?" "How much more could I take?" I was the sole provider in my household! How would I continue to pay for my prescriptions? How would I afford the co-pay for medical visits? Would I be able to put food on the table? This was a reality and I had to deal with it.

My emotions were naked and transparent. They had been stirred up! I was livid and upset! I had the right to be angry, scream, and to let off some steam! The anger had caused doubt and had already blurred my vision and thoughts. Negativity had seeped in; my thoughts were foggy, cloudy and warped.

The circumstances up to this point knocked me lifeless. I felt as if I was beaten to a pulp and tossed in mid-air. I felt as if I was spun around in a circle, then in an upward and downward motion, just like a leaf tossed in the wind. I felt as if the downward motion begun. I was in slow motion. My entire being was crippled. I lost coordination with my hands and feet. I plummeted into an abyss of fear. I was overcome with anger and panic which was not a good combination. It was nightfall! I was emotionally drained! I chose not to nurse my anger or give room to my fears. None of them was good for my health and wellness.

I fell on my knees and said my spiritual anthem, Psalm 121, *"I will lift up my eyes to the hills from whence cometh my help..."* My prayer was to remove the anger, the fear and darkness. "Lord, create in me a clean heart and renew a right spirit within me."

I knew that my future was in God's hands and I asked the Lord to give me total peace about my future. God is able! He answered my prayer and removed my anger and fear. Light had begun to break through. Ecclesiastes 11:7 says: *"Truly the light is sweet, and a pleasant thing it is for the eyes to behold the sun."*

Philippians 4:19 says, *"God will supply all my needs."* God knew what was best for me! My former job was stressful. The program that I was responsible for would be scrutinized from time to time by certain regulatory agencies who would conduct surveys. I had to ensure that verification of documentation was done in a timely fashion. I had to be knowledgeable on Bylaws, Rules and Regulations. There was no room for errors. There were deadlines attached to each function; monthly meetings, semi-annual meetings, and minutes developed from the meetings. I always had to be on point.

The stress would have been too much during chemotherapy. My body would hurt so much after the injections were administered; I am not sure whether or not I would be up to work. I now assume the stance that everything happened for the best.

Desperate Means called for Desperate Measures:
Miracle One

On June 15th, I went to the Department of Social Security and filed for disability. The application took some time. Someone told me that I would have to obtain a legal aid attorney to represent me, since the Department of Social Security does not always give approval the first time around. I was approved within two days. I knew the Lord was on my side.

I had been Side-Swiped twice but the quick approval from the Department was a Miracle! Payments would not begin any time soon. Nevertheless, I was grateful and thankful.

With a letter from the Department of Social Security, I went to the Medicaid offices for assistance. Bear in mind, I had no medical insurance; there were medical bills that were unpaid; I would still incur more bills with chemotherapy. I had nothing! Long story short, I was denied! The circumstances did not matter, I would have to be homeless, destitute and penniless to get assistance.

What Do I Do Now? My Ad

What was my next move? I had bills to pay but no income. Should I stand at a designated corner, where traffic is constantly flowing, hold up a card board written in my favorite color and in my best handwriting my ad would read:

- I am 63 with no income; Cancer in remission;

- I have a mortgage (not homeless yet)!

- No change too small!

- Can work – Got job?

Help! This is an everyday dilemma in the world! Forget the pride; Forget the stares; Forget you, if you think I am faking it; If you think I am making this up, Forget you! I am holding up my cardboard proudly' This is my Ad! Are you looking? Are you listening? Hi Mister, Hi Ma'am – I'm over here! Help! I Need Somebody Help!

Third Treatment (June 18th): Miracle Two

I prepared for chemotherapy like I usually do the night before. On the day of my appointment, I had to inform appropriate personnel at the Cancer Center check-in desk that my position was terminated. I no longer had an income or medical insurance. I prayed and then applied to the hospital for financial assistance. The medical bills were so exorbitant and would continue to be so.

Labs were done and I proceeded to the treatment area, settled in. The IV process went smoothly. I would be there for the usual five hours.

I was scheduled for an injection on June 19th. This time it would be administered once rather than in series of three. This type of injection is called Neulasta. It is a prescription medication called a white cell booster that helps the body produce more white blood cells to reduce the risk of infection.

Neulasta helps provide protection with one injection per cycle of chemotherapy. It is given 24 hours after chemotherapy is administered.

On the following day, I had a reaction to the injection. My entire body began to hurt. I felt as if a truck had run over my entire body. When I inhaled and exhaled my body hurt. I was on the sofa in a fetal position like a baby who needed to be picked up, cuddled, rocked and have a lullaby sung to me. The discomfort continued for two days. "Lord, help me to endure." There was not a lot of movement going on. Tylenol provided a little relief. I made a mental note to take the Tylenol before my next injection.

Approximately two weeks later, I received notification from the Cancer Center that my application for financial assistance was approved.

A great burden was lifted. I was so relieved. God had answered my prayers.

Other private practices extended 100% financial assistance. Others discounted their financial services. This was much appreciated. I was again grateful and thankful for another miracle. God is truly able, He is my shepherd, my provider and I shall not want. Thank you Lord.

In Between Treatments

My hair loss was continuing big time! It was happening all over my body. From the crown of my head to the soles of my feet! One day as I shampooed my hair and massaged my scalp, I heard Plop! Plop! Plop! I looked down and there was most of my hair in big clumps. I stood there for a while with the water running on my head and body. I looked at what had happened. I was in a state of shock. I looked in the mirror and stared at my head. It looked like someone had given me a Mohawk haircut! I just stared at it. When I snapped out of my shock, I asked Jason to shave the rest of the hair. He refused to do so. He said, "Mom, I just cannot do it." I borrowed his clippers and shaved off whatever hair was left on my head. I was now totally bald. My scalp was sore after my hair loss. The soreness did not last long.

That day, I was not angry. I was mentally and emotionally prepared for the day when my hair loss would happen. Instead, I was very quiet. I said, "Lord, it's just you and me!" There was something about the loss of my hair and the baldness! It was confirmation that I had cancer. Being bald, I still looked feminine. However, there was this innocence and vulnerability with my baldness that was evident.

I got my Bible and started to read the New Testament. I had to focus on healing. Matthew, Mark, Luke and John were all about miracles and healing by Jesus. I read it! I breathed it! I was focused! I claimed healing from the inside out. I read the New Testament in its entirety in six months.

Wig Happy

I was never a big fan of wigs. I had always admired them and liked them on others. So, I now dreaded the thought of wearing one, though I knew I needed it.

I started to cover my head with caps, bandanas and scarves. I thought about Jason's reaction to my baldness. He knew that my head was bald, but never saw it. I knew he was scared. I understood, and realized that it was a lot to deal with. One moment, I had lots of hair and suddenly there was none.

I had a conversation with him one day that I could not always cover my head. It was summertime and my head was hot and needed to breathe!

That weekend I came out and said, "Jason, this is what I look like, here I am!" He looked at me, hugged me and told me I was beautiful.

I went wig shopping and bought couple of wigs. They were long, short, spiky and curly wigs. I was wigged up! I would switch from one style to another so frequently that people did not know who I was. When they recognized me, I would chuckle on the comments they would make, such as, I liked your hair better in this style or that style.

Regardless of the compliments, I had to get used to the wigs.

Since it was the summertime, my head would be so hot! There were times I felt like yanking it off my head in public! At home I did not wear any wigs.

Acts of Kindness

Whatever the occasion, no one is under obligation or is compelled to give anyone anything or do something for them. So, when someone took the time to think about me I was thankful and grateful. I have learned not to say, "You shouldn't have!" Instead, I say "thank you."

During my journey with cancer, there were so many acts of kindness extended to me. One day, I was doing some quick food shopping. After collecting my items, I joined the line and awaited my turn to pay for my groceries on the counter. I got distracted talking to a neighbor. When I turned around my groceries were not on the counter, they were in my cart. The woman who was in front of me, said, "There you go," as she placed the last bag in my cart. I knew I had not paid for the groceries, and I wondered why they were bagged and in my cart.

I looked at the cashier. She said, "they have been paid for." The woman who was in front of me said, "I took care of them." Still a bit confused, I looked questioningly at her. She said that the Lord had placed it on her heart to pay for my groceries and she was obedient. I thanked her profusely for her act of kindness and, before I realized it I was in tears.

I followed her to the parking lot and thanked her again and again. We talked for a while. I told her that I was going through some health challenges. She asked for my name. She promised to pray for my healing and for me to cast my cares on the Lord. I shared the story with my son when I got home, and we both thanked the Lord.

On another occasion, I was shopping in the same super market. While in line someone came up behind me and put something in my hand. It was money from a friend of mine, I thanked her. She told me that she loved me and we hugged.

On another occasion, I had a sudden burst of energy and made the decision to clean my garage. With mask and gloves, I started to clean. A couple who lived in the area came by. They knew about the surgery, not the diagnosis of cancer. My head was covered with a bandana and was saturated with sweat. My face was dripping in sweat. Yet, they wanted us to hold hands and to pray. They showed no concern for my sweatiness.

I am thankful and grateful that Dr. G.I. my Gastroenterologist monitored my health issues and referred me for a CT Scan. I appreciate her commitment to patients. It is because of this commitment and persistence that my life has been spared. I applaud her commitment, dedication and quality care she provided to me.

I am thankful and grateful for the flowering plants, flowers and cards, from my former employer, friends and church family.

I am thankful and grateful for the donations from co-workers during my employment. This has not gone unnoticed, especially during a time of recession and reduced hours at work.

I am thankful and grateful for all the scrumptious meals that the Baitys' have fed me again and again. They have done much to satisfy my unusual cravings.

I am thankful and grateful for the home visits from Judith and her mother, Miss Cecelia. I would chuckle when they arrived announcing, "We are here to look for the sick and the shut-in."

I am thankful and grateful for the "Ensure" drinks, the Josephs' family bought for me.

I am thankful and grateful that the Josephs' family picked me up after the first chemotherapy.

I am thankful and grateful for the loaves of whole wheat bread the Gibbs' family gave me.

I am thankful and grateful for the phone calls from my family and friends.

I am thankful and grateful for the phone calls from friends who were aware of the surgery, not the diagnosis.

I am thankful and grateful that Miranda stayed the entire day at the hospital on the day of my surgery. I am thankful and grateful she held my hand.

I am thankful and grateful for my son and friends who visited me the night of my surgery.

I am thankful and grateful that Mary Jane spent the night at the hospital and massaged my feet when they were so cold.

I am thankful and grateful for all the prayers.

I am thankful and grateful that Evelyn, my grandson's Mother brought Jaylen to see me.

I am thankful and grateful for the monetary gift Evelyn surprised me with.

I am thankful and grateful that Christine, my sister, took vacation time, flew in from Connecticut to take care of me.

I am thankful and grateful that my cousins Angella who lives in Charlotte, North Carolina and Geneve who lives in New York visited with me.

I am thankful and grateful that Maria flew in from Florida to see me and encouraged me to journal my experiences. I am thankful and grateful for the inspirational books you gave me.

I am thankful and grateful that Julie and her husband, Alex, who lives in Florida, visited me. I am grateful and thankful for the gifts.

I am thankful and grateful for the Sour Sop leaves and "Complan" my sister, Jean gave me. Complan is a complete nutritional meal in a drink.

I am thankful and grateful for my inner circle and their strong support system throughout my journey.

I am thankful and eternally grateful for every demonstration of love that was shown in "Acts of Kindness."

My Two Sons

I love my sons Jason and Winston! There is a twenty year difference between them.

When Jason was conceived, I was 39 years old. The Lord knew what he was doing! I am so appreciative that throughout my illness, he was with me. Having Jason at that age allowed him to be still living with me. Although, he could have lived on campus, he chose to do the daily commute which is approximately one-hour roundtrip. He is my only family in the city where we live. I know he will leave one day, but in the meantime, I am grateful and thankful that he is here with me.

Jason is a full time student with a hectic schedule. He was always aware of whatever I was going through and was always tender and affectionate to me. He knew when I had good days and when I had not so good ones.

I knew he loved and trusted the Lord, however, when a loved one is diagnosed with a disease such as cancer, it is a very difficult experience. I reminded him that I was always available should he wished to talk about cancer, chemotherapy, anything that I had experienced or whatever he felt. I encouraged him to read the book of Job.

Job loved and feared the Lord and avoided evil. His body was covered with boils from head to toe. He was in pain. He lost everything - family and possessions. Job was at his lowest. Yet, he still feared the Lord.

Job 19:25-27, says, *"I know that my redeemer liveth, and that he shall stand at the latter day upon the earth; And, though after my skin worms destroy this body, yet in my flesh shall I see God. Whom I shall see for myself and mine eyes shall behold, and not another; though my reins be consumed within me."*

Job trusted God despite the problem. He knew that God was faithful and kept his promises. Job was not only hopeful, but he had faith, determination and patience. Have you ever heard the remark that says, "He or she has the patience of Job?" His patience was indeed rewarded. Job had a great ending and was even rewarded doubly for the things he lost.

Winston, my firstborn, who lives in New York, struggled with my illness. I believe the distance made it even harder for him to deal with it. This was the son, who sang to me on mother's day. He always, said, Mom, you are my favorite girl!" He does not hesitate to express his love for me.

My Mother helped me raise Winston. He was raised to love the Lord. The day I told him about the cancer, I felt as if I was marked for death. It seemed he had given up hope already. "You are my only Mother, I love you, what am I going to do?" he said. We spoke about the importance of thinking positively, not negatively.

That was the only time he spoke that way. He meant no harm. He may have forgotten for a quick minute that there was nothing too hard for the Lord, and that He was and is still in the healing business! With some encouragement from me, he was able to cope much better.

Fourth Treatment (July 9th)

I continued with the usual preparation for the fourth treatment. I had two more treatments and looked forward to the fifth and sixth treatment. That would be it!

On the day of my appointment, I did not look or feel any different this time. There was a connection with the patients who sat in the waiting room. Patients either showed their baldness, or covered their baldness. I was in the mix - my baldness was covered.

The nurse or "sticker" who usually administered the IV was retiring. This would be the last time she would administer the IV. I expressed my appreciation for everything she did for me and wished her well. Treatment that day went smoothly.

An injection (Neulasta) was scheduled for the next morning. This time, I took Tylenol in advance to minimize the after effects of the injection. It helped some. I was in bed or on the sofa, not doing much. This would last for no more than two days. I had to get used to the discomfort. The horrible metal taste in my mouth did not make me feel any better.

In Between Treatments

I had lost so much weight. I looked ok, but the weight loss was evident. The only signs of sickness in my body were the loss of my hair, weight loss, dryness of the skin and side effects from the injections, I was not sick. There was no diarrhea, constipation, vomiting or nausea. I often wondered whether or not the chemotherapy was working. I was assured that whether there were side effects or not, they do not determine how well the chemotherapy was fighting the cancer.

The cravings got worse. I tried to satisfy them as much as I could. It also meant that with the cravings, I would eat more. I usually ate small portions of food, about five to six small meals. a day. Even though I became a "picky" eater, I had a decent appetite most of the time. On days when I did not have much of an appetite, I drank Ensure or smoothies, which are high in protein and calories that my body needed.

My finger-nails were turning dark and were very unattractive looking. There was nothing that I could do about it. It was one of the side effects that I told myself, "It is what it is."

My eyebrows and eyelashes thinned out. I thought this was nothing compared to some of the patients who were extremely sick and required oxygen tanks, wheel-chairs and canes. I was grateful.

Fifth Treatment (July 30th)

My cousin, Angella knew that I was scheduled to have surgery in April. She was unaware that I was diagnosed with cancer. At the time that all of this was transpiring, her mom had passed and I chose not to tell her of my health challenges, since she was going through a lot with the loss of her mom.

In August she learned that I had cancer. She immediately came to visit with me and accompanied me to the Cancer Center for the fifth treatment.

This was the fifth treatment. I had just one more treatment. I was praising God. I went through the usual preparations for the treatment. I checked in at the registration desk. I completed my labs and I was on my way to the treatment area knowing it was almost over.

I requested a nurse or "sticker" who was good at finding a vein quickly. I got one and the IV process went smoothly. It was count down for me! I was very excited that this was my second to last treatment.

Since chemotherapy was a five-hour process, I do the treatments without someone accompanying me. My friends worked or had their own schedules. I had become accustomed to having this time alone. I forewarned my cousin that I was not much of a talker during and after chemotherapy. She did not mind. She just wanted to spend time with me.

She came bearing gifts: already cooked soup – this was no ordinary soup. It was a combination of lentils, green split peas and butter beans. The soup was delicious. She also made "corn meal pudding" a dessert which I had not eaten in many years.

She shared lots of family stories that I did not know about. The stories were funny. She brought lots of family photos, black and white photos. Each photo had a story. During her stay, there was a lot of laughter. I shared with her that her visit was at the right time and much appreciated. It was great to have her spend some time with me.

I looked around at the familiar faces in the treatment room. Some were not there. I wondered if they had completed their chemotherapy and the cancer had gone into remission. I wondered at their outcome?

There were new faces too. This meant they were those who were beginning their new cycle(s) of chemotherapy.

An injection (Neulasta) was scheduled for the next day. I took Tylenol prior to the injection to minimize the pain. I still experienced some discomfort and the horrible metal taste in my mouth. As usual I would rest and not do much for the weekend. Angella stayed the weekend with me.

There were times she would have an expression of sadness. We were going to church and I had put on a wig. This was the first time she saw me in a wig. She "teared" up for a bit. I told her that I was at a good place and that it was well with my soul.

Her husband, Ira, came to pick her up. Before they left, he prayed and asked the Lord to heal me from the inside out! That was a prayer from the heart. There are some people that can pray. They are not timid to pray in public. When they are through with prayer, you want to say a loud "Amen and Amen."

Just before leaving, Angella asked for a group hug. It was so precious. I really love my family.

Chemotherapy can cause damage to the nervous system. Many of those damages could get better within a year of the completion of chemotherapy. Some could last the rest of someone's life.

Some of the nervous system damages began to become noticeable. I developed muscle weakness in my left leg. I often felt as if my leg would buckle. There was also soreness around the hip area. I also became tired more quickly and there were times that I was actually out of breath and would sweat profusely when I climbed the stairs in my home. I became very concerned about these side effects. I informed my physician. She consoled me with the information that these were the expected side effects from the chemotherapy drug (s).

Sixth Treatment (August 20th) and Reflections

This was the last and final treatment. Sound the trumpet! The night before I did the usual preparation for the treatment. I swallowed the pills with ease. I could not wait for daybreak!

The usual registration check-in was done. Labs were done. I proceeded to the treatment area and announced, "This was my last treatment." The IV process went smoothly.

I was in a bed and a private room this time. I reflected on my journey so far. I was so ready for this treatment to be over.

The back of my hands were sore, swollen, and black and blue due to the insertion of the needle for the IV. I had to use compressors on both hands from time to time. The skin and the veins on the back of my hands were extremely dark. I was told that my natural skin tone would return after I had completed all of my chemotherapy.

Most of my finger-nails were totally dark, especially on my right hand. My eyebrows and eyelashes had fallen off. These areas were totally hairless! The Lord blessed me with long and beautiful eyelashes. There was never a need for me to enhance my eyelashes. Hopefully the re-growth would be the same long and beautiful eyelashes I had before chemotherapy.

I certainly would not miss the pills that I had to take the night before and at 3:00 A.M. the morning of the treatments.

My journey began in December 2009. I thought about the medical professionals who provided quality care throughout my treatment. I was very fortunate and blessed to have had such wonderful human beings around me: To my Internal Medicine physician, Gastroenterologist, Obstetrician and Gynecologist, Oncologists, Anesthesiologist and the nurses (stickers) in the treatment area, many thanks for the quality care you provided to me. If I were asked to complete a survey on patient satisfaction, it would be: Very satisfied.

I was also grateful to the CNAs, front office admission staff, and administrative staff for being so professional and polite. A special thank you to the employee from housekeeping who diligently performed her job duties during my four-day hospitalization.

I appreciated the volunteers who were dedicated and committed to help sick people. I made a mental note to look into the volunteer services after my chemotherapy. I would like to give back! All of my memories were good ones.

My treatment ended, I was on my way home. I sang, prayed and praised the Lord for his goodness. There were no injections scheduled for the next day.

August 30th – Doctor's Appointment

Ten days after my last treatment I had a doctors appointment. The usual labs were done and reviewed by the physician. I was scheduled for an injection. I requested the series of three (Neupogen) instead of the one-time injection (Neulasta). I preferred

Neupogen, since the side effects would be more bearable.

I was told by my physician that a CT Scan was scheduled in September. An appointment was made for me to see the Oncologist for a checkup. I was told that the results of the CT Scan would be discussed at that appointment.

I received the great news that the CA-125 was now within the normal range. My progress looked great! I knew the Lord was working it out!

September 13th (Day of CT Scan) and My Mortality

In preparation for the CT Scan, I drank a creamy/chalky/vanilla like drink in advance.

The CT Scan was done in the morning and went smoothly. I was confident and at peace with my journey.

I was at a crossroad – a busy intersection of my life. Do I turn left or right? Do I go straight or make a u-turn? I did what I knew best to do. Pray. I prayed, "Lord, put me on the path you want me to be." "Please give me total peace about the results, whatever it may be."

Have you ever heard the expressions, "Here today, gone tomorrow," or "Life is too short?" I am often reminded of those expressions when someone dies – whether it was a family member, close friend, or a co-worker. Perhaps it was the tragic death of someone I heard on the news who I may not even know. Nevertheless it made me sorrowful and sad.

The expressions, here today and gone tomorrow or life is too short, made me think of my mortality. In my opinion it meant that tomorrow is not promised to me. The expressions became more real to me with a life threatening disease.

If tomorrow is not promised to me, "Now what?" "Do I change?" When do I change?" or "What do I change?" The answer was a resounding, yes to I have to change and change now.

I developed a *Nora List* keeping in mind that I am work in progress. This meant that my list was not final, but rather a starting point.

1. Keep God first in my life

2. Surrender all to God

3. Stay spiritually fed

4. Nourish my body with God's word

5. Be appreciative and grateful for a new day

6. Live each day as it was my last

7. Detoxify my heart, soul and mind

8. Have a clean heart and new spirit

9. Forgive myself and others who may have wronged me

10. Learn from my mistakes

11. Let go of the past and move forward

12. Do not let my past hold me hostage

13. Do not stress

14. Learn how to be at peace and be calm

15. Avoid confrontation

16. Resolve issues immediately

17. Do not go to bed angry

18. Do not sweat the small stuff

19. Love my family - Tell them that I do

20. Appreciate friendship

21. Help, encourage and inspire someone

When I lay down to sleep at night, I am at peace. When I live to see another day, I am at peace.

Got Hair?

Soon after my last chemotherapy, my scalp turned dark. I thought my scalp was dirty. I looked closely at my scalp and realized that the hair was growing back and had made its way to the surface. This was followed by "stubble" on my scalp, which felt prickly. "Stubble" turned into "fuzz," which turned into jet black soft hair – just like a newborn baby. There was a touch of grey on the sides. The hair just laid flat on my head. Close to my ears on each side, there were patches of hair that were curly; a complete different texture from the rest of my hair. I was not sure how this new growth would turn out.

There was also growth on the other parts of my body that had had hair loss. I was very excited! This re-growth reminded me of what takes place in the spiritual realm. It speaks of rebirth and is reminiscent of David's admission that *"we are so fearfully and wonderfully made."* Psalm 139:14. Yes, we are so wonderfully created by the Almighty God. Like David, I will praise God for how I am made. Especially after cancer, *"my soul knows it right well."* Psalm 139:14.

I recalled that in February, I spoke to my hairstylist about the use of chemicals in my hair. I wanted to transform my hair into a natural look. At that time, my hours at work were reduced and a natural look would be more affordable.

Little did I know then that I would be diagnosed with cancer where the hair would fall out due to chemotherapy and my wish would come through? Cancer was a rough, tough and horrible process to obtain the natural look I wanted. I am quite sure that I will now be styling a natural low cut look.

September 15th (Visit with Oncologist): Miracle Three

I arrived for my appointment and was escorted to the Oncology section. I was told to undress and put on a gown. The doctor came in the room and we greeted each other. She made a comment that "I looked great, the CT Scan was fine, there were no issues and the cancer is in remission." My response was "I know!" even though I did not know anything! Those words came out of my mouth automatically without even thinking, and then I said, aloud – "Praise God."

The examination went well. I would be placed on a three month schedule for labs and to see the doctor going forward.

The National Cancer Institute's definition of remission on the web is "A decrease in or disappearance of signs and symptoms of cancer." In partial remission, some, but not all, signs and symptoms of cancer have disappeared. In complete remission, all signs and symptoms of cancer have disappeared, although cancer still may be in the body."I have claimed healing from the inside out.

As I was getting dressed, I began to say a prayer of thanksgiving. This was miracle #3.

Part III

Still Standing - Holy Ground Experience

A Holy Ground experience is not restricted to an edifice such as a church. It can happen anywhere. Moses had his holy ground experience near a burning bush where he was told to remove his shoes for the place where he stood was holy ground. God's presence is everywhere.

As I left the hospital and hurried towards my car, I could not explain what I felt or what happened in the hospital parking lot. I knew that I was sobbing while I was praying. I felt this peace throughout my being and knew that the presence of God had surround me right there in the hospital parking lot. It was as if I stood on Holy Ground.

I got into my car. My heart was full! Tears of joy trickled down my face! I first called my sons with the great news. I called my sister and my closest friends. I could not stop crying tears of joy. As I drove home, a song popped into my head. The title of the song was:

"Bless the Lord Oh my soul, and all that is within me, bless his holy name."

I recalled that the song is based on a scripture from the Bible. I could not wait to find it. When I got home, I dashed for my Bible and found the scripture in Psalms 103. I read all twenty-two verses.

Psalm 103:3-4 touched me and spoke to my spirit.

"Who [the Lord] forgiveth all my iniquities, and healeth all my diseases." My diseases!! How awesome! *"Who [the Lord] redeemeth my life*

from destruction; who [the Lord] crowneth me with loving-kindness and tender mercies."

I believe with all my heart the Holy Spirit put this song in my heart, which lead me to find where it was written in the Bible so that I would read the third and fourth verses. I knew that this was a confirmation from the Lord, that he never left me during my illness and he would never leave me nor forsake me. With his stripes, I was healed.

Psalm 103 is now my spiritual anthem of thanksgiving. I was so thankful, so grateful and yet excited at the same time. The rest of the day was quiet, alternating between tears, prayers and songs.

Jaylen is in The House

Jaylen, my seven year old grandson and Evelyn, his mother, visited with me. It was great to see them both. It was perfect timing since it was post chemotherapy. Other than my slimness and my baldness, I looked good and was excited to see them.

When I picked them up at the airport I had worn a wig. I did not want Jaylen to see my baldness. I was concerned that he would be scared or afraid of me. At home, I removed the wig and put on a bandana.

One day, Jaylen was upstairs and he looked over the banister and asked "Where is your hair, Nana?" I told him to come and sit with me so I could explain. I told him that I was sick and the doctors gave me medicine. It caused my hair to fall out. I also told him that I felt much better and my hair was growing back. He asked me to remove the bandana and I did. He looked at my head, rubbed it and said Mmmm!!! He did not seem bothered about my baldness and went about his business after that.

I was relieved that I did not have to wear a bandana for the duration of his visit. I learned later that Evelyn, his mother had a conversation with him about cancer and what happened to cancer patients.

My cousin, Geneve and her husband also came for a visit. They had vacationed in South Carolina and planned to stop by on their way back to New York. While they spent just one night, it was good to see them. It was great to see family!

Surprise Package

On November 4th, Maria, a dear friend of mine and one of Jason's godmothers, who lives in Florida, called. She said that someone who lived in Raleigh, North Carolina, would be in the Greensboro area and would deliver a package from her. A time was set for November 5th at 3:00 P.M. She gave me the name of the person who would deliver the package.

Sure enough at the appointed time someone drove up. We greeted each other. After some pleasantries, she stated that she had forgotten the package in the car, and had to get it. I stood at the door and awaited her return. Can you imagine my shock, surprise and joy when I saw Maria, my dear friend, walking up the walkway? Surprised and flabbergasted, I ran in the house and sobbed. Hugs and smooches followed. It was a wonderful moment; a fabulous surprise and a great visit.

I shared with her about my illness and my journey. She encouraged me to journal my experience. She also updated me on her family and grandchildren. Family really is everything!

It was a short visit indeed. However, I assured her that it was not how much time one spent with someone that mattered. What mattered most was the quality of the time that was spent.

In my busyness, I am so guilty for not keeping in touch with loved ones. Sometimes it takes a Side-Swiped situation to reconnect. It does not mean that I do not love or care for someone anymore, but, my busyness gets in the way and I lose touch. Have you ever felt that way too?

It was a wonderful thing in the case of the surprise visit from Maria, that while we had not spoken for a while or I did not let her know of my illness immediately, she understood. We talked as if I had seen her yesterday. We also knew that we were in each other's thoughts and our hearts.

When the Unexpected Happens – Can We Talk?

We all go through stuff at one time or another. None of us gets exempted. What matters is how we react to what happens and in whom we place our trust.

How many times, have we talked to our girlfriends, family members or guy-friends and we are told, "I have not seen or heard from you in a while?" The answer frequently given is, "I was going through a lot" or "I had some issues."

At times, life takes us through valleys, mountains and places so much that we do not know whether we are coming or going. Life is like that sometimes.

All of us experience the unexpected and the unplanned. We all have circumstances that we did not see coming. We have all been Side-Swiped!

Something happens when the planned becomes the unplanned and the expected becomes the unexpected. It does not matter how much of a planner one is, a panic button becomes activated at that particular time.

My first thought was to give up with the diagnosis of cancer and the termination of my job. My spiritual tank was tilting towards empty. I had to tap into and draw upon my inner strength to fill up my spiritual tank. Praise God, I am energized, I am rejuvenated. I am now the little engine that keeps chugging along, "I know I can."

When the unexpected happened to me, and the panic button activated, I did not beat myself up, I did not moan and groan and think "Woe is me." Reality kicked in and I had to figure out how to fix it. How do I get out of the rut? Of course, the great answer was taught me as a child by my mother, *"I can do all things through Christ which strengthens me."* Philippians 4:13.

My plan was to retire at age 66 and everything would go smoothly. It did not happen that way. I was 63 years old when my position was terminated, which meant, there would be no income for the next three years.

As a result, everything was affected such as my finances, my relationships and my health. The stress factor was there and everything became chaotic! It was not supposed to happen this way. My plans were ruined!

What about the stress factor? I had major surgery. Cancer was found in my abdomen. Chemotherapy took its toll. I lost my hair. My weight dropped significantly. My position/title was eliminated. The job is now done by other people. I had mortgage responsibilities and other expenses. Should I be stressed? Yes! Those Side-Swiped moments called for a hair pulling tantrum. Luckily, I did not have hair on my head to pull.

How did I minimize and manage the stress factor?

- I recognized that there will always be little and huge challenges in my life

- My wellness was very important to me

- I was always prayerful

- I asked the Lord to remove all my worries and give me peace

- I read the Bible frequently, especially portions of the Bible that was comforting

- I read inspirational books

- I surrounded myself with positive people

- My surroundings were tranquil and peaceful

- I treasured quietness in my alone time

- I rested

- I attended the mid-day services to receive a blessing

- I took the focus from me and direct it on others

- Inspired someone

- Helped someone

- I watched sitcoms that would make me laugh

- I changed my mindset

The Lord knew the beginning, the middle and what the end will be. Jeremiah 1:5, says, *"Before I formed you in the belly, Nora, I knew you. And before you came out of the womb, Nora, I sanctified you."* I have personalized this verse.

My mother when she was alive always told me that, "God will not give me more than I can bear." I believe the experiences we encounter are a part of God's plan. Perhaps it is to get our attention, or to polish and shine us up a little bit, and to remind us that He is in charge.

Sometimes, we will get so low in our lives, that we have no other choice but to have a fresh start in our relationship with the Lord as was the case with me. He is a God of chances, so that I, Nora can make things right.

When I was very young I established a checking account. This was my first checking account and was very inexperienced. I would get a notice in the mail from the bank to advise me that a check had bounced due to insufficient funds. I thought no way! I would spend hours, reconciling my bank statements or balancing the check book and go over each entry to see where my math was incorrect. The fees charged for insufficient funds would affect my budget.

After a while, I would take my time to ensure that the entries in the checkbook register were entered correctly and that the math was also correct.

So it is in my personal life. When I hit a pothole, I take inventory of my life to see where I am. Am I a debit or a credit?

Save for a Rainy Day

I always had a job. The job has been my partner for most of my life. The partnership lasted for many years. We had a lot going for us: stability and growth. There was a "Win-Win" situation with the job. The sensible thing to do when you have a job is to save for a rainy day and have a "nest-egg."

Whatever the financial goal, whether it is a 401K, money market, stocks and bonds or savings account, it is wise to save something. Small amounts of money turn into large amounts. Every little bit helps! Be committed and stick to the financial goals.

Whether or not you are a homeowner or you reside in an apartment, a Side-Swiped situation can happen at any time.

The situation will be minimized when there is a "nest-egg" for a rainy day.

My Health

As a young girl, the word cancer to me meant death. There was no hope, it was final! That was my mindset growing up.

Adults were afraid to say the word, cancer. It was called the Big C! At times, the word was spelt, not spoken. I had enough sense to know what the word was.

As I got older, I had concerns about diabetes since my dad had the disease and was on insulin all of his life. Diabetes was the cause of his death. There were other family members diagnosed with diabetes.

I would have vivid flashbacks as a child as I witnessed my dad injects himself with this needle. I did not know exactly what he was doing and dared not ask. Children were to be seen and not heard – therefore I kept within my allowable limits.

I remember that he would stick himself in the leg. He must have been nervous, since his legs would shake and in a child's mind, I could not comprehend what was going on. I knew for sure that this routine made me uncomfortable and fearful. Perhaps an explanation to me at the time would have been comforting.

As I got older, I understood what the injections were all about and had to educate myself on the disease.

Many years later l was diagnosed with Type-2 diabetes. I was not placed on insulin. I do recall when I was told that I had diabetes, I was extremely upset. It was the worst illness I ever had and I was even embarrassed to let anyone know of the diabetes.

The flashbacks returned to me as a child when my dad administered the injections and how his legs shook. My mind would play "tricks" on me and I would transform my thoughts where I administered the injections in my leg area. The power of the mind! It could make or break you!

It took some time for me to get over the diagnosis of the disease and the fear of dying from it. Now, I have accepted the diagnosis. I have also learned that it is managed with medication and diet.

My mother had cholesterol issues so I knew that I could be diagnosed with it. I was aware of the health issue when she passed. Later in my adult life high cholesterol was an issue and is managed with medication.

A change in my diet played a crucial part of my management with diabetes and high cholesterol.

With the diagnosis of peritoneal cancer, I did not lose my cool, I was very calm.

At one time, I thought I was in denial and perhaps would have to seek counseling.

I had to do a lot of soul searching and prioritized some things in my personal life. I had a different perspective and I began to view things differently. I never lost sleep, nor was I worried about the diagnosis of peritoneal cancer.

I noticed that early in the A.M. sometimes at 3:00 A.M. when all was still, I would just wake up naturally. I would talk to the Lord in silence, or listen to the Lord and things would become clearer to me. There are times that warm tears would flow, not because of sadness, but, just to think of the goodness of the Lord and how faithful He has been.

Early one morning, there was the still voice that reminded me I asked for peace no matter what the circumstance or situation I was going through.

At the age of 50, one of my requests to the Lord was for Him to give me peace, the kind of peace, that passeth all understanding. I prayed for peace, because of the turmoil, mayhem and drama-filled situations I went through. I was used to the turmoil, it was a part of my life. I thought it was normal. It was a process to switch from turmoil and experience the Lord's peace He wanted to give to me. God answered my prayer. I accepted this great and wonderful gift – Peace, which got me through tough times.

I realized that my reaction I had to cancer was the peace the Lord gave me. I am so thankful. It's a good place to be and I am grateful.

My Inner Circle

At the Education In-Service, we were told to avoid crowds of people and do less hugs and kisses during chemotherapy. This was necessary to avoid infections.

The Web's definition of "inner circle" is an exclusive circle of people with a common purpose. It was important for me to have people long distance or otherwise who loved me, who were positive, spiritual and who loved the Lord in my inner circle. I fed into that big time. It was a good thing for me.

There were families in the North Carolina area in my inner circle; my sons were a part of the inner circle. There were other family members and close friends who did not live close by who were a part of the inner circle. I had to make the decision regarding the "inner circle," because my health came first.

When I went to church, I would leave after the sermon, to avoid the hugs that I was accustomed to and actually even longed for but was unable to accept during my treatments. My health came first.

Negativity was not allowed. Negativity attracts anxiety, fear, anger and stress. The combination of these "weeds" is definitely not good. We cannot let the "weeds" turn into roots which can find their way in our minds and get embedded.

I do believe that God will hand pick people and place them when the time is right in your life to help you through challenges, from the lows to the highs. This has been the case with my inner circle.

Full Circle

Looking back, I believe with all my heart that I was prepared spiritually, mentally and emotionally for the cancer diagnosis and my journey about two years ago.

I was asked to be the music director (direct the choir) for my High School reunion in Montego Bay, Jamaica in 2007. The songs I selected for the choir was Faithful, Faithful is our God and Great is Thy Faithfulness.

On another occasion, it was placed on my heart to have a Women's Day program in my church. I coordinated the program with the Women's Ministry leader. The Holy Spirit had already placed on my heart the theme, the format for the entire day and the speaker. The theme was, *A Clean Heart and the Right Spirit*. The Women's Ministry leader was accepting of it. It was well attended and I believe it was a blessing.

I did a piano selection at a church in New York, when I visited my family during Christmas 2009. Led by the Holy Spirit, I played a medley of songs: My Peace, Total Praise and the Lord's Prayer.

Working with the youth in the church where I am a member, the songs selected had to do with the heart, peace, thanksgiving and faithfulness.

Whatever I felt in my heart was evident in the selection of songs or whatever the theme was. These wonderful experiences prepared me for my journey. My faith and trust in the Lord was solid and unshakeable.

Close Encounter with the Bible

During my journey, I selected scriptures from the Bible (King James Version) that became the source of my strength and gave me Peace. I have selected various verses. Please read the referenced verses in its entirety, if you can.

- Psalms 23 – *"The Lord is my Shepherd, I shall not want..."*

- Psalm 34 - *"I will bless the Lord at all times; his praise shall continually be in my mouth…"*

- Psalm 46 – *"God is our refuge and strength, a very present help in trouble…"*

- Psalm 51: 1-12 – *"Have mercy upon me, O God, according to thy loving kindness: according unto thy multitude of thy tender mercies blot out my transgressions..."*

- Psalms 103 – *"Bless the Lord, O my soul and all that is within me, bless his holy name. Bless the Lord, O my soul, and forget not all his benefits; Who forgiveth all thine iniquities; who healeth all thy diseases…"*

- Psalms 121 – *"I will lift up mine eyes unto the hills, from whence cometh my help. My help cometh from the Lord, which made heaven and earth…..."*

- Psalms 139 – *"O Lord, thou hast searched me, and known me. Thou knowest my downsitting and mine uprising, thou understandest my thought afar off…"*

- Psalms 145 – *"I will extol thee, my God, O King; and I will bless thy name forever and ever…"*

- Philippians 4:6-8 and 19 – *"Be careful for nothing; but in everything by prayer and supplication with thanksgiving let your requests be made known unto God…"*

- Isaiah 53:5 – *"But he was wounded for our transgressions, he was bruised for our iniquities: the chastisement of our peace was upon him; and with his stripes we are healed…"*

- Proverbs 3:5-6 – *"Trust in the Lord with all thine heart; and lean not unto thine own understanding. In all thy ways acknowledge him, and he shall direct thy paths…"*

- Matthew, Mark, Luke and John – Please read if you can about the miracles that were performed.

Jesus was and is still in the healing business – Miracles still happen and I am proof!

Songs of Inspiration

I grew up on hymns which have inspired me during my challenges or potholes in my life. It does not matter whether I am singing, humming or playing the piano. I have found comfort and peace in these songs. Some of these songs are ones that my mother used to hum. She hummed a lot. The titles of the songs are:

- I feel like going on

- It's so sweet to trust in Jesus

- I need thee every hour

- Oh the best friend to have is Jesus

- I need thee Precious Jesus

- I need thee every hour

- Precious Lord, Take My Hand

- My Peace

- All the way my Savior leads me

- Day by Day and with each passing moment, Strength I find to meet my trials here

- Great is thy Faithfulness

- Faithful, Faithful is our God

- Under his wings, I am safely abiding

- My Soul is anchored in the Lord

Sour Sop Fruit

The Sour Sop is a fruit. I grew up eating Sour Sop fruit and at times it was made into a drink! Yum!! What I did not know was that this fruit and the leaves were very medicinal and are used for medicinal purposes including cancer.

A friend of mine called to say that after the treatments that I should drink sour sop leaves as a tea or as refreshing cold drink. He e-mailed an article on Graviola Leaf. This is the same as the Sour Sop tree that is grown in the Caribbean.

I called my niece, Marcia to see whether or not she could find the leaves in Brooklyn. I was told that my sister, Jean, had two trees on her property in the Caribbean. I was so ecstatic! My sister who was in the Caribbean at the time dried the leaves and mailed them to me.

I now have my sour sop leaf tea to drink very frequently. I am a believer!

Be Careful How We Treat Others

In one of my former positions, there was a young woman who smoked and for some reason called me Auntie. While not knowing why, I saw it as a sign of respect, which, meant that I must have made some impression on her. I therefore accepted her as a niece and answered to it. It was a cordial, professional and respectful relationship.

I always encouraged her not to smoke! She would go on cigarette breaks and whenever she went on those breaks, I would be coming out of my office, walking down the corridor, or going for a walk. It never failed! She would smile and say, "Auntie, don't say a word, just pray for me."

Checking in at the Cancer Center and going through the admission process for outpatient services, I was pleasant and upbeat. I greeted everyone with respect even though I was going through my trials.

I later found out that the young woman who smoked and called me Auntie was related to a worker in the facility where I had chemotherapy. Moreover, this worker was one who assisted me with the outpatient process.

What if I was rude or judged the young woman who called me Auntie? What if I had not taken the time to speak words of encouragement to her? Even though it is the responsibility of her relative at the Cancer Center to treat everyone fairly, sometimes things are not always done fairly. There is a phrase that says, "What goes around comes around," or the golden rule that says, "Treat others as you want to be treated."

Who knew that our paths would cross? What this reinforces for me is that this is a small world that we are living in! It pays to be careful how we treat people!

Fruits of the Spirit

My Pastor recently talked about the Oil of Joy (Isaiah 61:3; Psalms 45:7). He said that when we have the Oil of joy, it improves our personality; it oozes a positive spirit; it dramatically increases our energy; it transforms our worship and carries us through tough times.

I am convinced that I had the Oil of Joy before my journey with cancer started in April 2010. It is because of this Oil of Joy that gave me peace to have endured so much. I Am Oiled Up! Lord, I thank you for the Oil of Joy.

I know for sure that the Lord had granted me peace. "Aren't joy and peace part of the Fruits of the Spirit?" "What happened to the other Fruits of the Spirit?" "Do I have them?" Galatians 5:22, says, *"But the fruit of the spirit is love, joy, peace, longsuffering, gentleness, goodness, faith, meekness and temperance."*

"Lord, you know that I am work in progress; please let all, not some of the Fruits of the Spirit live and stay deep in my heart, soul, mind and body. Let them be infused deep within my veins. Please clothe me with the Fruits of the Spirit."

Growing up, there was a song that we sang at church and in school. The words are very special which says:

"I have the joy, joy, joy, joy down in my heart, down in my heart to stay; I know the devil doesn't like it, but it's down in my heart, down in my heart to stay; I have the peace that passeth understanding down in my heart, down in my heart to stay..."

My Faith Journey

My journey is nothing more than a journey of faith. The American Heritage College Dictionary defines faith as confident belief in truth, value or trustworthiness of a person, an idea or a thing; A belief that does not rest in logical proof or material evidence.

- Hebrews 11:1 says, *"Now faith is the substance of things hoped for, the evidence of things not seen."*

- I had faith that *"I can do all things through Christ which strengtheneth me."* Philippians 4:13.

- I had faith that *"with his stripes, I am healed."* Isaiah 53:5.

- I had faith that God is still in the healing business.

Faith does not require a canister filled with mustard seeds in order for results to happen. We must believe that when we have faith as a grain of a mustard seed, obstacles and hurdles will disappear and diseases will be cured. Only a grain! Not much of a prerequisite for faith to work.

My life has not been a "bed of roses." There have been more potholes, bumps, detours and dead-end situations in my life which would qualify me as a candidate for a lifetime of counseling. Through it all I have learned to trust in Jesus, have faith, and believe that it will get better.

One day I was talking to my niece, Marcia about my journey. I told her that I was a late bloomer. I referred to myself as a late bloomer because I wrote Side-Swiped, my first book at age 63. Who would have thought that this would happen?

My niece reminded me that we are all on this train ride with lots of subway stops. We get off the train at what we think is our designated stop. Then, one day, the Lord will change our designated stop and place us at another destination, where our journey will begin on a new path.

She reminded me that all the Side-Swiped situations I experienced happened for a reason. They all caused me to realize that I have a talent that the Lord gave me.

So, here I am at the age of 63 a late bloomer with blossoms.

As I have aged, I have blossomed into a well rounded person who gained wisdom from all of the obstacles and hurdles that I experienced throughout my life. I am confident and happy. My heart, soul, mind and body survived the trials and when I look in the mirror I see this fine piece of art – Me! I am special!

What if you have faith and your circumstances have not changed? Things did not work out! "What then?"

"You don't look to the left or to the right – you continue to be faithful and keep your eyes steadfast on God."

When we are faced with challenges, we ponder the "what-ifs", we terrorize ourselves and place unnecessary pressure on ourselves and we lose focus.

This is when we are at our weakest and can become susceptible to the enemy's tactics. In my opinion, the enemy is the greatest schemer and strategist. He hides and waits for the opportunity to pounce on us.

We forget to exercise our faith and forget that we can cast all our cares on the Almighty God.

Praise God, the devil is defeated. He is evicted out of my life and has no part in it.

Isn't it sweet, though, that we eventually realize that we can cast our cares on God. We can hold up the white flag and say, "I surrender!" We can tell the Lord, all the sweet nothings: "I love You Lord, I trust You Lord, and I have faith in You."

God loves us with an unconditional love – no matter how many times we fall short. He welcomes us back into his arms; he tucks us under his humongous wings where we can safely abide forever. Isn't that awesome? I want to shout Hallelujah! Don't you?

When I was at my lowest with the diagnosis of cancer and the termination of my position during chemotherapy, it took courage on my part to take a leap of faith. Faith that God would make the impossible, possible and that He would heal me.

I have always prayed that my two sons would give their hearts to God. A pastor once referred to Isaiah 49: 24-25 in one of his sermons and stated that this was the scripture(s) to read and meditate upon should we desire that our children be saved.

"Will the prey be taken from the mighty, or the lawful captive delivered? But thus saith the Lord, Even the captives of the mighty shall be taken away, and the prey of the terrible shall be delivered: for I will contend with him that contendeth with thee, and I will save thy children."

Evangelistic meetings were scheduled to be held by my church. I read, prayed and meditated on the above scriptures every day. I prayed that Jason would accept the Lord as his personal Savior. I knew that it would happen. I just did not know when the Lord would do it!

Jason accepted the Lord in his life in November 2007. I had faith that the Lord would hear my petition. He did and I experienced one of the greatest joys that a parent could have. I treasure it.

I am still prayerful about Winston. We have frequent conversations about his relationship with the Lord and I have no doubt that he does have one. However, my prayer is for him to wave the white flag and surrender all to the Lord and not just have a relationship but an intimate relationship. I have faith that it will happen. At the end of the day, timing is everything. It's in God's time.

Once upon a time, I would just do my own thing and would not seek the Lord for guidance. I would make a "big mess" of things – all the time! It took most of my adult life to figure that out. So, whenever I have to make any decisions, I pray for guidance and wisdom and I wait to hear from the Lord.

God is the greatest director and producer there is. He sits high and looks low; He directs and guides me. I listen for "Action" or "Cut!." It is

God's timing, not mine. He is in charge! It's all about faith.

"For we walk by faith, not by sight." 2 Corinthians 5:7.

God is a global and a universal God. He is here, there and everywhere at the same time. He can multi-task more effectively and efficiently than anyone else can! He can fix anything, He is an amazing God.

My faith has been in God, not in man, my children or friends! It has found a resting place in God and God alone!

Renewed Commitment

I gave my heart to the Lord when I was eight years old. In my twenties, I drifted from the Lord, but, praise the Lord, he never left me. Throughout the years that I drifted, I still loved the Lord. The commitment was there it was just very wishy-washy! I still prayed, read the Bible and would go to church when I felt like it.

Later in my adult life, I rededicated my life to the Lord. I always loved the Lord and always had a close relationship with Him.

When I was diagnosed with type-2 diabetes and high cholesterol problems, I was prayerful. I was sincere in my prayers.

At one of the youth day programs held at my church, my son, Jason preached a mini-sermon on "Remove the Mask." Reveal who you are and stop the pretense.

When I was diagnosed with peritoneal cancer, everything changed! My perspective changed. I could not be the same person. Not that I was a bad person, I had to change from the inside out with a pressure washer cleansing. It was a cleansing that cleaned out the soot, impurities and residue of anything that did not belong in my being.

It took cancer to knock some sense into me and I removed the mask!

The Lord has my full attention now! I have a renewed commitment! He created in me a clean heart and renewed the right spirit within me.

Not only do I have a close relationship with God; I have an intimate relationship. This intimacy allows me to experience the power of God.

I am not ashamed to say that, There is nothing between me and the Savior. He is my all and there's nothing between.

A Love Connection with Nora

When I lived in New York, I was very guarded. I was cautious on the subway, at work and no one was allowed in my space. I had a barrier around me.

When I moved to North Carolina in 1998, I was in my front yard doing some gardening. As the cars sped by, the drivers would wave to me. I did not return the wave! I looked behind me to see whether or not someone was behind me. I was guarded.

In the grocery store, shoppers would greet me, "How are you today?" The shoppers would keep going. I did not respond. Again, I would look around me to see who they greeted. I was guarded.

I quickly realized and got used to the culture of North Carolina. The residents that I came into contact with were very polite, hospitable and warm people.

Perhaps these traits made it easy for them to be nice, and not guarded to a stranger. The demonstration of warmth was unusual to me. Was this a culture shock? Of course! Do I now do the same? Absolutely!

Living in North Carolina, I retrained my mind and have learnt not to be so busy. I have learnt to enjoy quality of life. I have let my guard down.

Diagnosed with cancer forced me to have a love connection with myself. My emotions have become transparent. I appreciate every day. It is not unusual for me to express my appreciation to someone. My inner love connection has spilled over to my sons, family members, friends and those who I am in contact with. It is not unusual for mc to "nod" my head to acknowledge someone in passing.

A love connection with me is a beautiful thing!

Prayers of Thanksgiving and Supplication
Conversations with My Father

Prior to my journey, during my journey and post my journey, I prayed a lot! Sometimes the prayers were brief, other times lengthy. The brief prayers would be like, "Thank you Lord," or "Help me Lord," or "I need you Lord." These were said in the car, while I was gardening, cleaning or in the supermarket.

The lengthy prayers are in the early mornings and at bedtime. I am never in a rush. I am having a conversation with my Father, my Daddy. In the stillness of the morning, the tears would warm my face as I am one on one with my Father.

I would always begin with the Lord's Prayer. After, the Lord's Prayer, my prayer would be as follows:

Thank You Lord for waking me up this morning to see a brand new day. Thank You Lord for grace and Your tender mercies towards me. I am thankful that You are my Redeemer, my Restorer, and my Shelter in the time of storm. You are my refuge and strength and a very present help in trouble. You are my Jehovah Jireh, my provider. I am thankful that You are my shepherd and I shall not want. I am thankful that You are my way in, my way through and my way out.

I am thankful that You are my healer and my greatest physician. Your word says that by Your stripes, I am healed. Father, I stand on Your word. I accept it, believe it, and claim it. Thank You for healing me from the inside out. I am thankful that You have given the doctors and caregivers the wisdom and knowledge to take care of me. I know that my steps are ordered by You, so I don't have to worry. I am thankful that You don't slumber and You watch my back, my side, and my front 24/7.

My future is in Your hands and I ask that You give me total peace about it. I am so thankful and grateful that you are my Father, my Daddy and I am Your daughter and You created me; I am thankful that You will never leave me or forsake me and that You will always take care of me. I am thankful for all the blessings You have bestowed upon me;

I thank you for the challenges and the potholes that have come my way. They have made me stronger and have ushered me closer in Your presence. I thank you for Your unconditional love, even when I mess up. Your word says to trust in You with all my heart and lean not unto my own understanding. I trust You. I know that You have already taken care of my medical insurance, my unemployment situation and my financial challenges Your word says that with thanksgiving and supplication that I should make my request known to You. I stand on Your words and Your promises;

Thank You for my children, my grandchild, and my extended family. Deliver them from the prey and save them. Thank You for family and friends. Protect and bless them. Thank You for giving me the green light to write this inspirational book. Thank You for the wisdom and knowledge You have imparted to me during the daytime and the wee hours of the morning. This book is written to Your honor and glory. May it bless and encourage someone to have a wonderful and intimate relationship with You.

I love You Lord. I magnify and glorify Your name and I give You all the praise, the honor and the glory. This is my prayer in Jesus name, Amen and Amen.

You see, I have been through some "things" and when I came out of those "things," I cannot be stingy in giving praise to the Lord. Call me deranged or crazy, I have to praise Him. It's a praise that comes from deep within my heart, my soul, a space that only the Lord occupies. I have to raise my hands and magnify His name, because He is worthy of my Praise.

"For I know the thoughts that I think toward you, Nora, thoughts of peace, and not of evil, to give you, Nora, an unexpected end." Jeremiah 29:11

"Jesus Christ the same yesterday, and to-day, and forever." Hebrews 13:8.

God is good, God is great, Miracles still happen! It is well with my soul.

Thy will be done - Dear Heavenly Father

It is because of Your providential leading why this inspirational book has been written. You gave me the GREEN LIGHT to write Side-Swiped. Each word is to Your Honor and Glory. I dedicate this book to You.

Father, while I do not know who You will put in my path to get this inspirational book published, I know You do. I know that You will reveal it to me in Your time.

I trust You. I thank You in advance. Your will be done.

Your daughter,

Nora

Definitions

Biopsy: The removal of a small piece of living tissue from an organ or part of the body for microscopic examination. Biopsy is an important means of diagnosing cancer from examination of a fragment of tumor.

Colonoscopy: A procedure for examining the interior of the entire colon and rectum using a flexible illuminated fiberoptic instrument (colonoscope) introduced through the anus and guided up the colon by a combination of visual and X-ray control. During a colonoscopy specimens can be obtained for microscope examination using flexible forceps passed through the colonoscope and to remove polyps.

Carcinoma: Any cancer that arises in epithelium, the tissue that lines the external and internal organs of the body.

Colostomy: A surgical operation in which a part of the colon is brought through the abdominal wall in order to drain or decompress the intestine. The part of the colon chosen depends on the site of the obstruction.

Excise: To cut out tissue, an organ, or a tumor from the body.

Gastroenterologist: Physician who specializes in the study of gastrointestinal organs and their diseases, which include diseases of any part of the digestive tract and also of the liver, pancreas, etc.

Hysterectomy: A surgery to remove a woman's uterus. It may be done through an incision in either the abdomen or the vagina. During a hysterectomy, other female organs may be removed.

Helicobacter pylori AKA H-Pylori: The bacteria responsible for most ulcers and many cases of stomach inflammation. The bacteria can weaken the protective coating of the stomach, allowing digestive juices to irritate the sensitive stomach lining.

Intraperitoneal: Within the peritoneal cavity, the area that contain the abdominal organs.

Mesentery: A double layer of peritoneum attaching the stomach, small intestine, pancreas, spleen, and other abdominal organs to the posterior wall of the abdomen. It contains blood and lymph vessels and nerves supplying these organs.

Morphology: Refers to the size, shape and structure rather than the function of a given organ.

Omental fat: A sheet of fat that is covered by the peritoneum. The greater omentum is attached to the bottom edge of the stomach and hangs down in front of the intestines. Its other edge is attached to the transverse colon. The lesser omentum is attached to the top edge of the stomach, ad extends to the undersurface of the liver.

Oncology: Branch of medicine concerned with tumors, including study of their development, diagnosis, treatment and prevention.

Oncologist: A board certified medical specialist who specializes in management of patients with malignant diseases, or treating cancer. Oncologists may be surgical (surgeons), clinical (experts in radiotherapy) or medical (experts in drug treatments).

Paracolic gutters: Spaces between the colon and abdominal walls.

Peritoneum: The membrane that lines the abdominal cavity and covers most of the abdominal organs.

Peritoneal serous carcinoma: A rare peritoneal cancer which involves the ovaries.

Polyp: A growth, usually protruding from a mucous membrane. Polyps are commonly found in nose. Other sites of occurrence include the ear, the stomach, and the colon.

Renal cyst: Small to large masses that grows on one or both kidneys.

Strandings: Small masses which can be seen with certain type of cancer that like to spread throughout the abdomen, e.g. ovarian.

Urinary Tract Infection (UTI): A bacterial infection that affects any part of the urinary tract. Symptoms include frequent feeling and/or need to urinate.

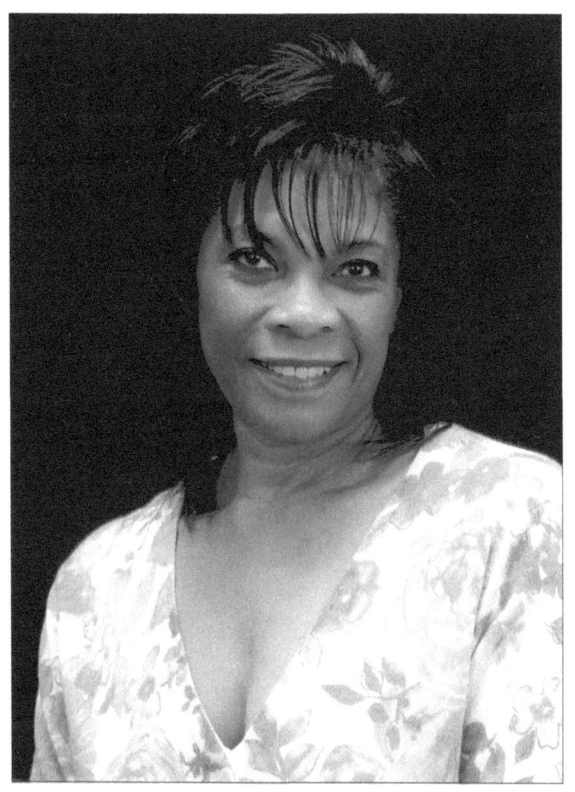

Photo before cancer -

Photo courtesy of Portrait Innovations.

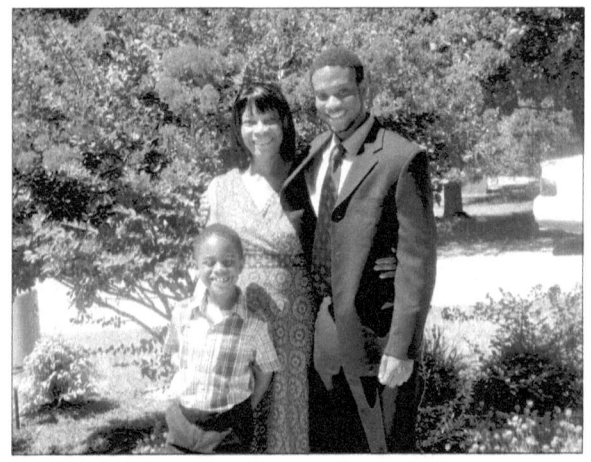

Photo with me in one of my wigs with son, Jason
and grandson, Jaylen.

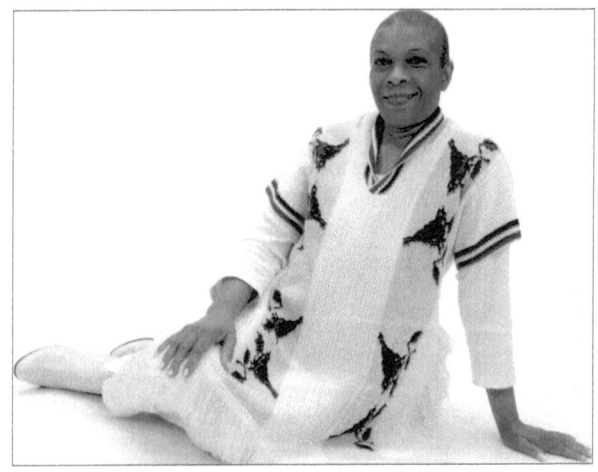

Three months after final chemotherapy -
Photo courtesy of Portrait Innovations.

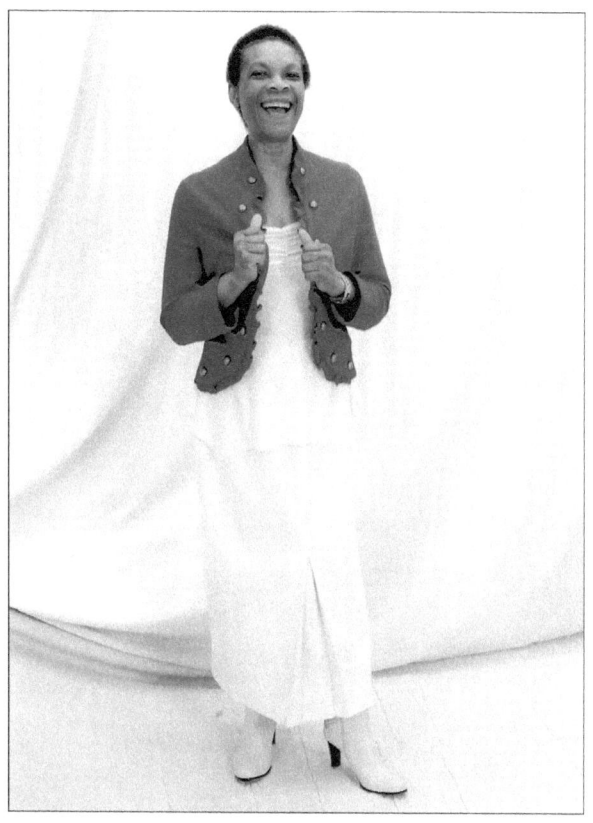

Seven months after final chemotherapy -

Photo courtesy of Portrait Innovations.

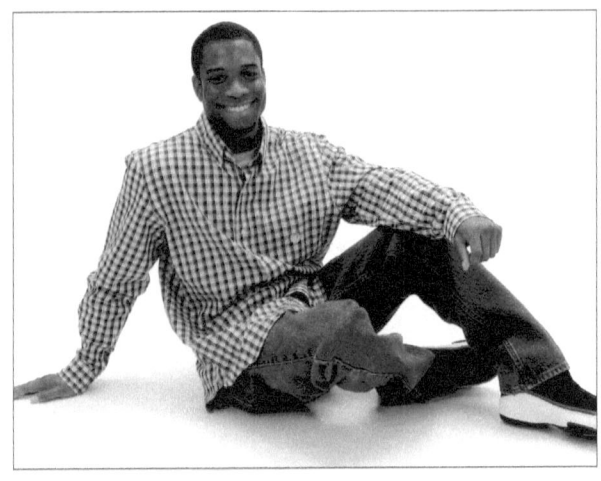

Son, Jason - Photo courtesy of Portrait Innovations.

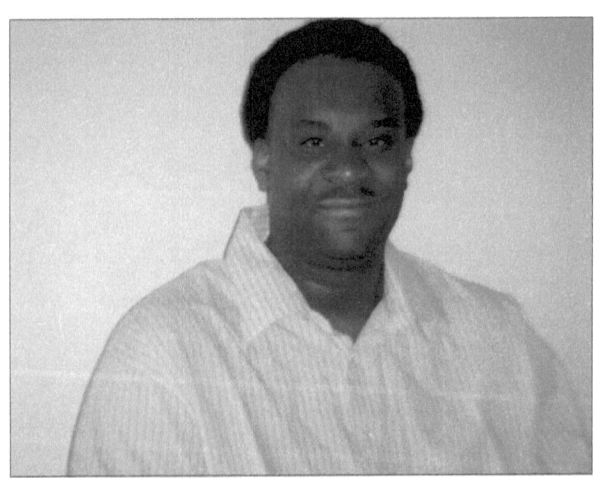

Son, Winston.

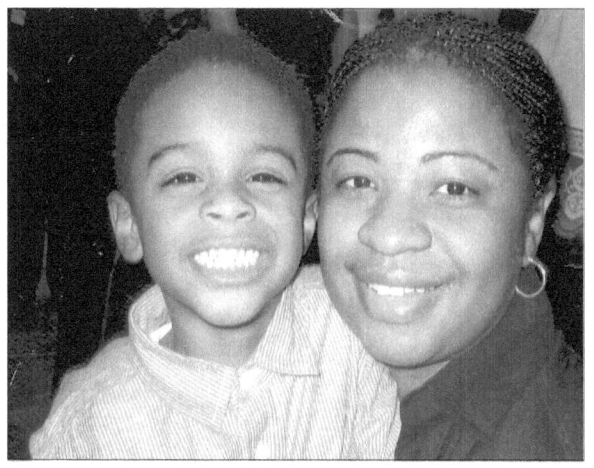

Jaylen, my grandson and Evelyn, his Mom.